D0245232

What Are You Really Eating?

How to Become Label-Savvy

AMANDA URSELL

HAY HOUSE
Australia – Canada – Hong Kong
South Africa – United Kingdom – United States

Published and distributed in the United Kingdom by
Hay House UK Ltd, Unit 62, Canalot Studios, 222 Kensal Rd,
London W10 5BN. Tel.: (44) 20 8962 1230; Fax: (44) 20 8962 1239.
www.hayhouse.co.uk

Published and distributed in Australia by
Hay House Australia Ltd, 18/36 Ralph St, Alexandria NSW 2015.
Tel.: (61) 2 9669 4299; Fax: (61) 2 9669 4144.
www.hayhouse.com.au

Published and distributed in the Republic of South Africa by
Hay House SA (Pty), Ltd, PO Box 990, Witkoppen 2068.
Tel./Fax: (27)11 706 6612. orders@psdprom.co.za

Distributed in Canada by
Raincoast, 9050 Shaughnessy St, Vancouver, BC V6P 6E5.
Tel.: (1) 604 323 7100; Fax: (1) 604 323 2600

A catalogue record for this book is available from the British Library.

ISBN 1-4019-0688-5

Printed and bound in Great Britain by TJ International Ltd.

For Geráld and Nana

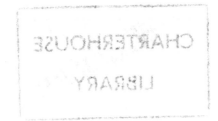

Contents

Acknowledgements

I would like to thank Michelle Pilley, Megan Slyfield and Jo Lal, at Hay House, who are a delight and revelation to work with. Thank you too to the wonderful Dr Beckie Long, a fab nutritionist and friend, who both helped me with some of the book research and read my proofs. Labelling is a complex issue and I appreciated your expert eye and encouraging words. I hope that Elliot, your little boy, was not too bored by listening to you read the proofs to him out loud!

1

Getting Label-savvy

If you have ever felt confused by the amount of information crammed onto a food label, then you are not alone and this is definitely the book for you. I'll let you into a secret – I'm a nutritionist and until I sat down to write this book, even I was bemused by some of the things I read.

When trying to make sense of labels it is first important to understand that they are there for two main reasons. From a practical point of view, they tell us the name of the food or drink we have picked up, which ingredients it is made from, its weight and where it comes from.

But labels are also there to encourage us to buy the product. They are like miniature adverts for themselves. It is their job to look as attractive and seductive as possible. The makers of foods and drinks do this by using bright colours and pictures, clever graphics and increasingly, these days, by highlighting their nutritional and health credentials.

By law, nothing on a food label is supposed to be misleading; however, at the moment, many claims about the nutritional or health benefits of a product occupy a rather grey legal area. Makers of foods and drinks stick, or are supposed to stick, to a set of voluntary guidelines. While in theory most of them do this, they also tend to make the most of their products' good points, while avoiding drawing attention to their less than virtuous ones. I suppose it is no different to anyone trying to make the most of their assets.

Making the most of themselves

I always think that labels are a bit like our clothes and make-up. We try to buy clothes that suit us and to wear make-up and do our hair in ways that enhance our good points. Similarly, if the maker of, for example, a biscuit knows that his product is high in fibre, he will want to tell you this on his label. This is essentially not that different to us wanting to make the most of having legs like Julia Roberts, if we are lucky enough to possess them, or a waist as nipped-in as Nigella Lawson's.

However, although the biscuit label might have a special flash saying 'High in Fibre', the manufacturer would be a bit bonkers if he were also to draw our attention to the fact that his biscuits are also packed with fat, sugar and salt. Not highlighting these points, which are obviously going to deter many customers from buying the biscuits, is rather like not wearing something that you know is going to accentuate those bits of your body you would rather play down. Just as most of us know how to dress to disguise these things, food and drink manufacturers know how to disguise the worst features of their products and show them in their most appealing light.

You cannot blame them. They are in the business of selling food and drink, after all, and want us to buy as much as possible. And, for now, it is legal for them to market their foods in this way. But understanding why and how manufacturers do this is important if you really want to get to the nitty-gritty of what you are eating.

Going back to basics

With between 20 and 30,000 foods and drinks now on sale in an average supermarket, learning how to read a label will help to put you in charge of your trolley when shopping, and allow you to make informed choices about what you, and others in your home, eat and drink.

My Nana, who is now 96, tells me that in 'her' day all food shopping involved a daily trip to local stores. To the baker for fresh bread made on his premises from scratch. To the greengrocer who popped carrots into a trusty string bag, and to the butcher who hand-wrapped a favourite cut of meat that was just enough for that night's dinner.

Today, we lead busy lives that mean we tend to do all our shopping in one go, under one roof in one supermarket, on a weekly or even monthly basis. Our shopping habits have changed; no longer do many of us walk around our local village or town buying bits and bobs from various specialized stores on a daily basis. Now we buy in bulk, and this means that most of the items we buy have in some way been processed before appearing on the supermarket's shelves. And since these foods come in packets, boxes, cans and bottles, it is just as well that, by law, they have to have a label. Labels on food have become a necessity.

What Are You Really Eating? is here to help you make sense of these labels, to give you the chance to really understand what you are feeding yourself and those around you.

So, what's on a label?

Labels may appear to be very different in shape and size, colour and design, and in what they tell us about the food or drink inside. But there are some things that are common to all labels that legally must appear.

For countries that belong to the European Union, like the UK, ultimately it is a group of bigwigs in Brussels who decide the laws that cover the labelling of their food. That said, here in the UK it is an organization called the Food Standards Agency who, in practice, handle things from a national perspective.

The key to tackling your shopping now and in the future is first to learn how to read the label. Then, perhaps most importantly, to learn how to interpret it. That means understanding, on the one hand, the information a manufacturer has to tell you by law, and on the other, the information he wants you to receive to encourage you to buy his product, rather than a similar one sitting right by its side.

Looking to the future

The powers that be over in Brussels are currently looking into various aspects of food labelling and there could be some changes in the next few years. The kind of areas being looked into for possible change include:

- the type of claims allowed to be made about the nutrients in food and their health value;

- how the presence of genetically modified substances in foods is flagged up.

These changes will be a good thing, but it means that the amount of information packed onto labels is going to increase even more.

Designing your own label

One way to get a good idea of what has to go on a food or drink label is to imagine designing one of your own. Let's say that you have just created your own range of pasta sauces and you have decided to call it 'Getting Saucy'. Okay, it's a terrible name, but bear with me! The first creation in your range is a great spicy sauce for pouring over pasta twists. Of course, you can't just make the sauce, bung it in a bottle and then ring a supermarket and ask them to put it on their shelves. One of the first things you will have to do is design a label. And there is a certain amount of information that our UK labelling laws absolutely insist that you put on it.

Its name

To begin with, you would need to decide on the name of your pasta sauce. How about 'Getting Saucy – The Spicy One'?

You could also give a little description right after the name, such as: 'A delicious sauce to spice up your life!'

What's in it?

Next, you would need to list the ingredients that you have used to make your new sauce. For example: onions, garlic, chillies, basil, tomatoes, plus any additives, such as preservatives, you have used to ensure the sauce lasts between the time it is made and the time your customers get to eat it.

But you cannot just write the ingredients down in any old order. You need to list them clearly and visibly and in order of descending weight. In other words, the first ingredient is the one the product contains most of. So your ingredients label could, for example, look like this:

Ingredients: Tomatoes, water, onions, garlic, basil, chillies, salt.

Its weight

Next, you would need to let your customer know how much your jar of pasta sauce weighed. For example, it could be a 400g jar. You could give this weight in imperial measurements too, if you like, but legally you do not have to.

When to use by

You would then need to tell your customers when your sauce should be used by and whether it needs to be stored in any special way once they get it home. For example, it may need to be stored in the refrigerator and used within two days of being opened.

Who you are

You would also have to put on your label the name and address of the people who make, package or sell the sauce. For example, you might have had your sauce made in Manchester. Putting the details of who made it and where means that customers can contact you should they have a complaint, comment or query. You never know, they may just want to write to tell you what a fabulous sauce you have concocted.

Special instructions

As if that was not enough information to have to squeeze onto your label, you would also need to let your customers know if there were any special things they had to do in order to use your product. In the case of your pasta sauce there would probably be no special instructions, although you would have to give the necessary instructions on how to use it. These could go along the lines of:

'Empty contents into a saucepan, warm through on a medium heat while stirring constantly for five minutes, and then pour over freshly cooked and drained spaghetti.'

Has it been treated in a special way?

You would also have to tell your customers if your spaghetti sauce had undergone any special type of treatment, such as ultra-heat treatment, or if it had been freeze-dried, concentrated or smoked.

Getting down to details

Those are the basics. If you want to go into more detail on your label, then read on ...

Listing ingredients

- Ingredients are listed in their weight-descending order at the time the product is being prepared.
- Water is listed in order of its weight in the finished product, although if it does not exceed more than 5 per cent of the finished product, producers do not need to bother telling you it is in there.
- When a product uses a variety of ingredients, such as herbs, but all in roughly the same quantity, then they can appear in any old order.
- In some cases the quantity of an ingredient has to be given on the label. For example, if you buy pork sausages, the list of ingredients must state the percentage of pork in the sausage. If a food emphasizes an ingredient by using a picture on a pack – for instance, if an apple pie has big pictures of an apple on the box – the ingredients label must give the percentage of apple actually present.
- With these and a few other exceptions, on the whole,

declaring the actual quantity of an ingredient in a product is not a legal requirement, although consumer bodies are hoping that one day it will be.

When ingredients do not appear –
the 25 per cent rule

- At the moment, there is a clause within ingredient listing called the '25 per cent rule'. For example, imagine that in addition to your range of pasta sauces you also made pepperoni pizzas. If a piece of pepperoni on a pizza makes up less than 25 per cent of your finished pizza, the ingredients in the pepperoni sausage do not need to appear on your pack. Which means that the pepperoni could contain colourings or preservatives and you would not have a clue that you were eating them.

- Another example would be if you bought a chicken tikka masala ready-made meal that contained curry powder. The curry powder would be less than 25 per cent of the finished dish, so the maker would not need to tell you exactly which spices he has used. Which means, for instance, that you will not know if any of the spices used in the curry powder have come from genetically modified crops or if they have been treated by irradiation.

Additives

- The makers of foods and drinks do need to let us know if flavourings have been added to perk up the taste of their products. So, if you had flung a bit of monosodium glutamate into your pasta sauce you would need to put it in the ingredients list clearly, telling your customers that it was a flavouring agent.

- Other additives also have to be listed, along with their main role in the food or drink. If you had added a splash of colouring to make your pasta sauce a deeper, more appetizing red, you would need to list its chemical name, or its 'E' number. (*Check out Chapter 13 to get a really good grip on additives, which ones are benign and which ones may be best for some people to avoid.*)

Pesticides, hormones and veterinary medicines

- Food and drink makers do not have to tell customers about any substances that may have been used in the processing or treatment of a plant crop or animal which appears in the final product. This means you would not have to mention on the label any pesticides sprayed on those lovely Sicilian tomatoes you've used, or any chemicals that stopped an ingredient, like the onions, from sprouting during its storage.
- Also, if your sauce contained meat, you would not need to inform people on the label of any residues of veterinary medicines that might be present. Which, of course, is one of the reasons why some people choose organic foods. The rules governing organic food mean they are open about any substances used and keep them to an absolute minimum. (*Check out Chapter 10 on Organic Food to find out more.*)

Foods that don't need a list of ingredients

- If you had decided to go into business selling fruit and vegetables rather than pasta sauces, then as long as you sold them whole and did not peel or chop them up into pieces, you would not have to bother with a label.
- The same is true of carbonated mineral water. As long as the bottle tells you somewhere that the water is carbonated, there is no need for a special little ingredient box saying: 'Water, carbon dioxide'.
- Vinegar, which has no added ingredients, does not need a list of ingredients.
- Even though flour has vitamins and minerals added by law, which is a practice that has hung over from the Second World War, when flour was fortified with these nutrients to improve the health of the nation, the packet only has to say 'flour' under the ingredients section.

Where does my food come from?

The country where a product underwent its last treatment or process is considered by law to be its 'country of origin'. Recently, the Food Standards Agency has said that if the ingredients come from a different place to this last place of processing, then we need to be told this on the pack.

For example, if ready-to-eat chicken drumsticks are cooked and packed in the UK but the actual chicken came from Thailand, the pack should say, 'Made in Britain from Thai chicken'.

Bodies such as the Consumers' Association, who are lobbying for clearer labelling, would like to see all foods carrying details of which country a food originally comes from. If it contains lots of ingredients from different countries, then it should say this, and at least try to narrow down where they came from.

Makers of foods and drinks cannot give their food or drink a name that implies it comes from a special place if it actually does not. You could not call it a 'Parisian Croissant' if your croissant was actually made in London.

However, there are exceptions to this rule, which involve well-known names of products that do not come from the place their names suggest. For example, Swiss Rolls do not have to come from Switzerland and Bakewell Tarts do not have to have been made in Bakewell in Derbyshire.

What's in a date?

Some foods have a date by which we are advised to use them. This is called a 'use by' date and it is put on foods like yoghurts and fresh meat which go off quite rapidly and, if eaten after that time, could quickly become a danger to our health.

The 'use by' date gives you a day, month and year by which the product should be used, along with specific details of the way in which the food must be stored.

In order to minimize the risk of going down with food poisoning, it is really important that we make sure these perishable foods are quickly taken from the shop and stored in the appropriate way, and then eaten before this 'use by' date runs out.

For foods that are not perishable, like packets of pasta or biscuits, boxes of breakfast cereal and cans of drinks, a 'best before' stamp appears on the label. The idea is that if you store the product as the label suggests (sometimes these details appear elsewhere on the product and not on the label itself), the food or drink will retain its properties until that time.

Obviously, just as in the old days of shopping, loose fruit and vegetables, fresh bread and foods like freshly baked scones and croissants that you buy from bakeries, do not have these 'use by' and 'best before' stamps. Neither, and perhaps less obviously, do foods like chewing gum, salt and vinegar.

Extra label essentials

- If a food like a pre-packed salad has been packed using a specially permitted gas, then the packet will tell you that it has been packed in a protective atmosphere.

- When the intense sweetener aspartame, whose brand name is *Nutrasweet*, is used in a food, drink or chewing gum, then the manufacturer also has to make a note that the product 'contains a source of phenylalanine'. This is a type of amino acid, or protein building block from which the sweetener is made, which is harmful to people with an inherited condition called phenylketonuria. These people can only tolerate very controlled amounts on a daily basis.

I am what I am – or am I?

- A label must tell things how they are. In legal terms, this means that it is illegal to mislead us as to the 'nature or substance or quality of the food', through the use of words or pictures on the label.

- It is a crime, therefore, for a label to tell us, or to imply with lots of pictures of big floppy sunflower plants, that we are buying sunflower oil when in fact the bottle contains a mix of sunflower and other oils, like rapeseed oil.

- It is illegal to pad foods out, for example, by adding cheaper cuts of meat to a meat pie that tells you that it contains premium steak. Or for manufacturers not to let us know that a food such as prawn, which we think we are buying fresh from the fish counter, has been previously frozen.

- Misinformation is at best bad news, because we end up paying more for cheaper versions of a product, and at worst a potential danger to some people's health. If, for example, a food has been filled with flour to make it go further and you suffer from gluten intolerance, then you could have an adverse reaction to the food. This is one of the many reasons why it is crucial for labels to be truthful.

When is a raspberry yoghurt not a raspberry yoghurt?

This might seem like a pretty straightforward question, but in fact you would need to know a few of the labelling loopholes to get the answer right.

For example, if you go and buy a 'raspberry flavour' yoghurt, you could be forgiven for thinking that the yoghurt

cont.

contains raspberries and that therefore you are upping your daily fruit intake by tucking in. In fact, a raspberry *flavour* yoghurt does not need to have been anywhere near one of these delicious little red berries. Flavour means just that: the yoghurt contains raspberry flavour, which is synthetic.

If, on the other hand, your yoghurt was described as 'raspberry flavoured', the raspberry taste would, by law, have to come mostly from real raspberries, although it would not actually need to contain whole raspberries.

Now you know!

- 'Flavour' means the flavour comes from additives – natural or synthetic.

- 'Flavoured' means flavoured with the real thing.

A picture tells a thousand words

There are also rules about the pictures that can appear on labels. The 'raspberry flavour' yoghurt cannot, for example, have a picture of raspberries on its pot, for the simple reason that it does not contain any. Raspberry-flavoured yoghurt, on the other hand, could.

Although this distinction is clear, sometimes pictures on packs can be a bit misleading. Take a 'Fruit Flapjack' that I bought recently. At least a quarter of the pack was covered in a photo of an oaty-looking flapjack bar, simply bursting with

raisins and cherries. A quick glance left me with the impression
from the name and the photo that this flapjack was a healthy,
fruit-packed choice. Yet when I got down to the nitty-gritty
and cast my eyes over the ingredients on the label I found that
it read:

'Oats, golden syrup, raisins, demerara sugar, hydrogenated
vegetable oil, vegetable oil, wholemeal flour, honey, dates,
cherries, sultanas, apricots, passion fruit, emulsifier.'

Sure, it contained bits of fruit, but with the exception of the
raisins, they were right at the end of the ingredient list, and
compared to the oats, syrup, sugar, oil, flour and honey the
flapjack contained, they were nutritionally insignificant. It was
a classic example of a pack implying it is one thing while being
another: what you got was probably not quite what a glance at
the label would lead you to expect.

But back to your pasta sauce ...

In addition to the information which you are absolutely legally
obliged to supply for your customers, there are other bits and
bobs you can add and it is up to you whether or not to include
them. Remember that in real life makers of foods and drinks
usually add other information to their labels with a view to
encouraging us, as shoppers, to reach up and put their product,
rather than a competitor's, in our trolley.

So, what further information might you put on your
'Getting Saucy – The Spicy One' pasta sauce, to show it in its
best possible light and persuade customers to buy it?

Further information

- If you think it would show your sauce in a good light, you could provide details about the nutrients that your pasta sauce contains. You are not legally obliged to do this, the choice is yours. If it has been made from gallons of oil and is really high in fat, you may decide not to.

- To help your customers put this nutritional information into perspective, you could also provide a little box of guidelines on the recommended daily amounts of nutrients for adults, so that they can compare the amount in the sauce to the total daily amount considered sensible for an adult man or woman. This, again, is optional.

- If, for example, your sauce is especially low in fat, you could splash a 'Low Fat' flash across the label. However, if you make any mention like this of its nutritional benefits, then legally you must provide a box in which the nutrients are listed.

- If you fancied it – and, of course, if it were true – you could also decide to tell your customers that your sauce was free from certain substances that might trigger allergic reactions in certain people. Like the fact that it is wheat-free, for instance. This would be useful information for anyone following a wheat-free diet.

- You could, although you do not have to by law, tell your customers about special methods used in the production of your sauce. Perhaps, for example, you had oven-roasted your tomatoes to extract every last scrap of flavour.

- If you really wanted to push the boat out, you could also

choose to give more details about how to use the sauce and maybe even provide a little recipe.

- You could add information about exactly where your ingredients came from to make the sauce look appetizing and authentic – perhaps saying that your tomatoes were grown and harvested from the sun-drenched isle of Sicily, for instance. This would conjure up all sorts of warm images that might just sway your customer to give your sauce a try.

- And if there is any room left, you may even decide to put a logo on your label. One telling you, for example, that your sauce is suitable for vegetarians. Of course you would first have to jump through all the hoops required to get permission from the Vegetarian Society to use their 'V' symbol, but if it boosted sales, then it may well be worth it.

Logos and endorsements

Labels often carry logos and endorsements. You might have seen a 'Tooth Friendly' logo on sugar-free packets of sweets, or the 'Soil Association' endorsement on a box of organic biscuits. If you would like to know how products have managed to get endorsements from organizations like the Vegetarian Society, and other groups like the National Osteoporosis Society, then there is a chapter on this later in the book (see Chapter 8). This explains what these logos mean, how a product qualifies for a logo or endorsement, and if they should really be influencing your decision in the supermarket aisles.

Comforting names

Products bearing words on labels like 'Handmade'; 'Authentic'; 'Home-made'; 'Hand-Reared'; 'Traditional' and 'Pure' will naturally make you feel cosy and warm because they are real 'feel-good' words. But what do they actually mean? In some cases not very much! (*Turn to Chapter 7 to find out more.*)

And finally ...

 Remember that labels are there to help you to decide which foods and drinks to buy. Knowing how to read the label allows you to discover what is really in these foods, how they compare to similar products and how they stand up on grounds of quality and healthiness.

 With all the thousands of foods and drinks just dying to leap into your shopping basket, learning how to read the label will really help you to take control over what you put into your cupboard, refrigerator and freezer – and ultimately what you put into your body and the bodies of those close to you.

 Be aware that it is completely natural for manufacturers to make the most of their products' assets, and that they will always tend to flag up their good points while playing down the 'bad' ones.

 If you want to make a comment or have a query about a label on a food or drink, you can always contact the company, whose details will be listed on the label.

2

Nutrition Labels

Flip a packet of food over, turn a bottle around, and more often than not, somewhere you will find a bunch of figures telling you how much energy and how many nutrients the food or drink inside contains. This is known as the *nutrition label*, and the decision as to whether to supply this information, or not, is down to the maker of the food or drink.

Taking the plunge

Those who do take the plunge to tell us the nutritional content of their product cannot pick and choose what they want us to know. If they want to mention the amount of energy it supplies, they must also tell us how much protein, carbohydrate and fat it provides per 100 grams.

This type of nutritional information labelling is known in the food world as 'The Big 4'. Don't be put off by the rather formal-sounding description – you will have seen it loads of times on everything, from packets of crisps and biscuits to ready-made meals and yoghurts.

'The Big 4'

'The Big 4' is the minimum amount of nutritional information that a manufacturer can tell us about their product. It must be given in the order shown below and be given per 100 grams (100g) if it is solid, for example bread or chocolate, or per 100 millilitres (100ml) if it is a liquid, such as orange juice or milk.

Typical Values per 100g (100ml)

Energy	kJ / kcal
Protein	g
Carbohydrate	g
Fat	g

What does 'The Big 4' label mean?

Energy, protein, carbohydrate and fat. We have all seen these nutrition labels often enough. But do we actually know what 'energy' means, or what on earth 'protein' is for? And even if we do – how do we know how much is enough, how much is too much, or how much we should be eating of it each day? If you have ever wondered any of these things, then the next section explains it all.

Energy

The energy a food provides our body with is measured in 'kilo-calories', which tends to be shortened and just called 'calories'. You cannot see 'a calorie' and calories are not a nutrient. They are simply the way in which we measure the amount of energy present in a food – just as we measure electrical energy in 'watts'.

It is the protein, carbohydrate, fat and alcohol in foods and drinks that actually contain, and therefore provide our bodies with, this energy.

What is energy for?

We need energy to fuel every single living process in our bodies. It fuels everything from the automatic beating of our hearts to the deliberate use of our muscles when we walk, run or jump.

What is a 'kJ'?

In the metric system, energy is measured in 'kilojoules', or 'kJ' for short. Because we are part of the European Union these also have to be given on the label, although most of us have not got the faintest idea what a kilojoule is.

If you do want to know, then here goes – one calorie is equal to 4.2 kilojoules. This means that if you ever find yourself in a European country like France or Italy and are just confronted by 'kJ' on a label, then you roughly have to divide the kilojoules by four to get an idea of the calories the product supplies.

How much energy do we need?

There is no getting away from it. If we consume too much energy in the food and drink we eat, then the excess is just converted into fat and shunted off to be stored in our fat cells. Which means that we end up gaining weight.

If you wish to lose weight you need to eat less energy. It's not rocket science! Becoming aware of the energy content of different foods and drinks by checking out the nutrition label is a good place to start when cutting back in order to shed the excess pounds. Keep reading to find out more about daily energy needs.

Protein

Protein is a nutrient and ensuring that we have a certain amount each day is crucial to our well-being. The word comes from the Greek *proteus* and means 'of first quality'.

Foods like meat, chicken, turkey, fish, eggs, milk, lentils and soy-bean curd (tofu) all contain lots of protein. Protein is made up from chains of building blocks called amino acids. Thankfully, labels do not have to tell us exactly which amino acids are in the specific food or drink but must only give us the total amount of protein, which is expressed in grams and appears on the label as 'g'. Once chewed, swallowed and digested, protein provides us not just with amino acids but also with energy.

Every gram of protein provides four calories. The amount of protein in a very lean 6oz (150g) steak is 40g (almost a whole day's needs), and it supplies 327 calories, most of which comes from protein. The energy from the protein in the steak is used to fuel cells. This means that the amino acids are taken off to maintain and grow new cells throughout our bodies, from all those in our muscles and skin to the cells that make our hair and nails. How much protein we need is mentioned later in this chapter.

Carbohydrate

Carbohydrate means 'carbon plus water'. Carbohydrates are basically compounds made by plants when they have access to water and are exposed to rays of sunlight.

Carbohydrates come in starchy forms, like rice and flour which is made from wheat, as well as sugary forms. Whichever form they start off in our foods, all carbohydrates, whether starchy or sugary, are ultimately digested into the simplest form of carbohydrate, such as glucose, which is the energy currency of every cell. Like protein, carbohydrates supply us with energy. Again, like protein, the amount is four calories per gram of carbohydrate.

Depending on which type we eat, carbohydrate foods also supply a range of other nutrients.

- An orange, for example, gives us 37 calories, most of which come from fruit sugar. It also provides practically our whole day's requirement of vitamin C.
- Bread gives us calories from its starchy carbohydrate – 77 calories in an average slice – plus B vitamins naturally present in the wheat from which the flour was made.
- Table sugar (sucrose), on the other hand, simply gives us energy and contains no nutrients.

On 'The Big 4' nutrition label all of these forms of carbohydrate are added together and given as one big total. No differentiation is made between whether they come from starches or sugars.

Fat

Strictly speaking, fats belong to a group of compounds that scientists call lipids. When liquid at room temperature, fats are known as oils, such as the sunflower oil we cook with and the olive oil we use in salad dressings. When solid at room temperature, they are just referred to as fats. Solid fats include things like butter and margarine.

For the purposes of 'The Big 4' nutrition label, all fats and oils are listed under the umbrella word 'fat' and given in grams. Fats are a very concentrated source of energy. Unlike protein and carbohydrate, they supply nine calories per gram – which is why fatty foods are so 'calorific'. The small amount of butter or margarine you put on a slice of bread, for example, has at least 60 calories, while the much bigger slice of bread has just ten calories more.

The Big 4 plus Little 4 Label

You have probably seen these four bits of nutrition information on your food labels many, many times. But the powers that be who deal with UK labelling laws would much rather manufacturers went the whole hog and gave us more in-depth information. This is found on what is known as the 'Big 4 plus Little 4' style of nutrition label.

In practice, this means that the nutrition label also tells us how much of the carbohydrate comes from sugar, how much of the fat comes from saturated fat, and how much fibre and sodium the food or drink supplies.

Although providing us with this extra information is generally done on a voluntary basis by manufacturers, there are instances when they must provide it. For example, if a manufacturer flags up on their pack that their product, for instance a packet of wholemeal fruit scones, is 'A Source of Fibre' or 'Low in Saturated Fat', then legally they must automatically give us 'The Big 4 plus Little 4' nutrition information as a matter of course.

What Does 'The Big 4 plus Little 4' Nutrition Label Look Like?

Per 100g or 100ml	
Energy	kJ / kcal
Protein	g
Carbohydrate	g
Of which:	
– sugars	g
Fat	g
Of which:	
– saturates	g
Fibre	g
Sodium	g

What does this extra information mean?

Sugars

The carbohydrate figure is the total amount of carbohydrate a food or drink contains, which includes starchy and sugary versions. This is why underneath 'carbohydrate' you can find the words ' ... of which sugars'.

Starches are the main forms in which plants store the energy that they need to grow and reproduce. Starches are long chains of sugars bonded together like the beads on a necklace. You find starches in grains of wheat and rice, and in foods made from these grains like bread, breakfast cereals and rice cakes. Starchy vegetables, like potatoes, are also rich in starch.

Sugars in food can come from those naturally present in the food, like those in fruit and sugar. But there are lots of added versions of sugars too, which you may have seen on ingredients labels. They include:

- Sucrose
- Glucose
- Glucose syrup
- Golden syrup
- Maple syrup
- Treacle
- Fruit juices
- Invert sugar
- Honey
- Fructose
- Dextrose
- Maltose

Under the word 'sugars' on a food label, there could actually be included any of these, as well as fruit sugar. However, it does not include the sugar from milk, which is called lactose. If you look at the nutrition label of a breakfast cereal, such as a '100 per cent shredded wheat' type of product, you will find that it contains no sugar. On the other hand, a sugary-tasting breakfast cereal, like a frosted flake cereal, does.

Saturated fats

All fats are made up from building blocks known as 'fatty acids' and fatty acids can come in three forms. You have probably seen these many times on food labels as you are going around the supermarket – they are saturated, monounsaturated and polyunsaturated fatty acids.

All fats, whether butter, margarine or olive oil, are a mix of all three fatty acids. What tends to happen, however, is that these different foods contain different proportions of fatty acids. Butter, for example, is made up of 62 per cent saturated fat, 30 per cent monounsaturated and 5 per cent polyunsaturated fat. Because the highest proportion of fatty acids are saturated, butter is referred to as a 'saturated' fat. See Table 1 on page 32.

On 'The Big 4 plus Little 4' label the total amount of fat is given in grams, plus the number of these total grams that are specifically supplied by saturated fat. The amount of saturated fat in a food is referred to on the nutrition label under the total grams of fats in the section that says 'of which saturates – '. Saturated fats have the effect of raising cholesterol in the blood, which may in turn increase our risk of heart disease.

Fibre

Fibre is also listed on 'The Big 4 plus Little 4' nutrition label. Fibre refers to dietary fibre, which is a type of carbohydrate. There are two types of fibre. One is 'soluble', such as the pectin found in apples and pears. It helps to slow down digestion and reduce cholesterol levels. The other, the 'insoluble' fibre, such as the fibrous husks in cereal grain, cannot be broken down by our digestive systems.

Unlike animals such as horses and sheep, for example, which have special digestive juices to break these tough 'fibrous' parts of plant material down and then absorb them for energy, in us they bulk up our stools and pass undigested out of our bodies. This insoluble fibre appears to reduce our risk of colon cancer and constipation.

Fibre is not found in animal foods like fish and meat but in plant foods like vegetables and fruits, and cereal foods like wheat and oats. The total amount of fibre in a food, including both soluble and insoluble, is expressed on the nutrition label as grams.

Sodium

Last but not least comes sodium, a trace mineral that we eat in very small amounts in things like sodium bicarbonate in baking powder, and the flavour enhancer monosodium glutamate. But these sources of sodium are tiny compared to the amounts eaten as 'sodium chloride', which is better known simply as salt.

On a nutrition label the amount of sodium appears in grams, or 'g'. On some labels the amount of salt (sodium chloride) is also provided and this is also given in grams. Because salt consists of two minerals, sodium and chloride, to convert the amount of sodium in foods into grams of salt you need to multiply by 2.5. For example: 1g of sodium = 2.5g of salt. It is hoped that before too long just the salt figure will appear on labels. Giving both sodium and salt levels is pretty confusing for most of us.

And there's more ...

As well as 'The Big 4 plus Little 4' a manufacturer can, if there is any room left on the label, go into yet more detail about the nutritional content of the product. This includes:

■ the exact amount of starch the product supplies;

■ the breakdown of the monounsaturated and polyunsaturated fats;

■ the amount of cholesterol present;

■ vitamins and minerals, if the product supplies significant amounts.

If the manufacturer makes any reference to these nutrients on the label, then the product must supply details of them.

What does this mean?

Starches

As well as giving the amount of carbohydrate in the product that is made up of sugar, the amount supplied by starches can also be declared on the nutritional label. This information absolutely must be given if the manufacturer has decided to draw our attention to the fact that the food is, for example, 'Low in Starch'.

Monosaturates and polyunsaturates

Similarly, if there is any mention on the label of the monounsaturated or polyunsaturated fats that the food contains – for example, a margarine boasting that it is 'rich in polyunsaturated fats' – then it must give the specific amount of polyunsaturated fats. The same goes for monounsaturated fats. (See also Table 1.)

Table 1 Type of fat

Type of fat	Satur-ated fat (%)	Mono-unsaturated fat (%)	Poly-unsaturated fat (%)	Known as
Olive oil	14	74	9	Monounsaturated
Rapeseed oil	8	59	32	Monounsaturated
Sunflower oil	12	22	66	Polyunsaturated
Soybean oil	9	23	51	Polyunsaturated
Butter	62	30	5	Saturated
Palm oil	47	44	9	Saturated

Cholesterol

If a label has splashed over it that its product is 'low in cholesterol', then the nutrition label must also tell you how much cholesterol the food or drink contains. Most of the cholesterol that circulates in our blood is made in the liver from saturated fats. Some foods, however, like eggs and cheese, cream and fatty bits of meat also contain ready-made cholesterol. These do not raise blood cholesterol.

Vitamins and minerals

Vitamins and minerals are 'micro-nutrients'. This means that you only need 'micro' (very small) amounts of them. This is why they are either measured in:

- milligrams, or 'mg', which are a thousandth of a gram. Vitamin C, for example, is measured in milligrams;
- micrograms, or 'μg', which is even smaller – one-thousandth of a milligram. Vitamin D and B12, for instance, are measured in micrograms.

Recommended daily amounts

The European Union has set down Recommended Daily Amounts for vitamins and minerals. The world of nutrition is littered with abbreviations so these are often just known as 'RDAs'. Recommended Daily Amounts are estimates of the amount of vitamins and minerals sufficient to meet, or more than meet, the needs of groups of adults.

For a food or drink to be allowed to mention that it contains a vitamin or mineral on its label, it must supply at least 15 per cent of the RDA for this vitamin or mineral per 100g, or per 100ml.

The Future

Trans fats

'Trans' fat are found naturally in minuscule amounts of meat and dairy foods; under natural circumstances, we would normally consume around 0.5g of trans fats a day. However, nowadays, we eat an average of 5g – that's one teaspoon a day, most of which is coming from margarine-style fats used in food production.

To make butter, milk is churned. Nothing is added, except a little salt. It is a natural process that has taken place for thousands of years. To make margarine, however, hydrogen is pumped through vegetable oil to change it from a liquid state to a solid one at room temperature. It is during this process that trans fats are created.

Research shows was that while saturated fats do some potential damage by raising our 'bad' low-density lipoprotein cholesterol, known simply as LDL (which sticks to artery walls and restricts blood flow), trans fats are not only capable of raising LDL cholesterol, but can also lower the beneficial high-density lipoprotein (HDL) cholesterol (which protects us from heart disease). This means that trans fats are likely to be even more harmful than saturated fats when it comes to increasing our risk of cardiac problems and stroke.

High intakes of trans fats have also been linked to the development of age-onset diabetes. Not only that: unlike 'good' fats like Omega 3s found in oily fish and nuts, which help to send messages between the junctions of nerve cells in the brain, trans fats seem to get incorporated into these junctions and once in situ block nerve transmissions. This means that they are in effect squatting in brain cells and disrupting the normal messaging services. Some scientists link the rise in the amount of trans fats in our diet over the last 30 years to the increase we are seeing in the number of dyslexic and hyperactive children.

In January 2006 trans fats will also have to be listed on nutritional labels in the USA. This is not yet planned in the UK. To reduce yours and your family's consumption of trans fats you need to avoid foods containing 'hydrogenated' or 'partially hydrogenated' fats on the ingredients list.

Putting this nutrition information into context

It is all very well being told how much energy, or how much of this and that nutrient, a product supplies per 100g or 100ml. But what is the point of providing this information if we do not know how much of these things we need and whether a food or drink is providing a little or a lot of them? Surveys on shoppers have shown that what we need is extra information so that these figures actually mean something.

For instance, say a food supplies 500 calories per serving, is that a lot or a little? How many calories are you supposed to have a day? A typical cheddar cheese has 22g of saturated fat per 100g. What does that mean to you and me? Is that a whole day's recommended intake of saturated fat or can we still have more from other foods? What amount constitutes too much saturated fat and, anyway, what happens if you have too much?

Some manufacturers are listening to the pleas of shoppers and have already begun to give us the extra details to make sense of the nutrition figures, but they are doing it on a voluntary basis. So have a good read of this information and you will start to see the wood from the trees and make sense of nutritional labelling.

Guideline daily amounts

Guideline daily amounts (yes, you guessed it, also known as 'GDAs') for energy, fat and saturated fats show the amounts suitable for average adults over eighteen who are of a normal healthy weight. They are beginning to appear on some labels but here they are so that you have them anyway. (See Table 2.)

Calories and nutrients per serving

In addition to the GDAs, research shows that we as customers would really like to see the nutrition information given per serving, which makes perfect sense when you think about it. What is the point of giving the amount of energy per 100g of a ready-made meal such as, for instance, lasagne, if in real life what you are sitting down to eat is a 350g serving?

Obviously, you could get your calculator out in the supermarket aisle and start trying to do calculations to work it out yourself, but that is a bit of a 'faff', isn't it. How much more

Table 2 Guideline daily amounts

Each Day	Women	Men
Energy	2,000 calories	2,500 calories
Fat	70g	95g
Saturates	20g	30g

Although no GDA figures have actually yet been given for protein, carbohydrate, fibre and sodium, here is a guide based on recommended intakes to give you an idea of levels to aim for:

Each Day	Women	Men
Protein	45g	56g
Carbohydrate	250g	313g
Of which sugar	28g	34g
Sodium	2.5g	2.5g
Salt	5.0g	7.0g
Fibre	18g	18g

useful then if manufacturers did the sums for us. If it is not possible, due to shortage of space for them to provide us with a full-blown set of figures per serving, then at the very least research shows that we would find it useful to have a little box telling us the energy and fat per serving.

For example, if a soup gave all of its nutritional credentials per 100ml, it could then supply a box underneath stating:

Per Serving (half a carton, 250ml):
85 calories   5g fat

The 'per serving' measure needs to be relevant to the product, for instance 'per slice' of bread, 'per biscuit', or if it is jam, 'per teaspoon'.

Some makers of foods and drinks are putting this information on their labels already. If it is not there, then at least you can become aware of roughly how much a serving is and do some rough sums to give you an idea of its total calories and fat content.

'High', 'medium' and 'low' nutrient levels

Another way of making nutritional information relevant would be if, as shoppers, we knew whether the nutrient levels in a food or drink are 'high', 'medium' or 'low'. If a sandwich supplies 20g of fat per 100g, is that a lot or a little? If it gives us 1g of sodium, is that high or low?

Giving us this information on the pack would allow us to put the product in context quickly and simply. It may be that in the future manufacturers will have to supply this kind of information but at the moment, once again, whether they do so or not is up to them. And to be fair, on some products there is precious little room to do so. So it is a good idea to keep in mind the information in Table 3. You can use it when shopping to give you a quick 'at a glance' idea of just how the nutritional land lies.

Table 3 Nutrient levels (*The amounts given are all per 100g*)

	High (a lot)	Low (a little)
Sugars	10g	2g
Fat	20g	3g
Saturates	5g	1g
Fibre	3g	0.5g
Sodium	0.5g	0.1g

The 'Traffic Light' System

The Food Standards Agency (FSA) is currently investigating ways of labelling food that will make it easier for people to choose a healthy diet. The method the FSA is most likely to adopt is the 'traffic light system'. This is because after much research with consumers, they found that the most popular system is the use of 'green', 'amber' and 'red' round symbols on foods and drinks, showing at a glance whether a food is OK to eat regularly, in moderation or only occasionally.

Two systems are being investigated:

- The first uses a green, amber or red symbol next to each nutrient on the nutrition information panel on pack. This would make it easy to see if a food or drink is high, medium or low in nutrients such as fat, sugar and salt.
- The second method would be to just award a single green,

amber or red symbol for the product as a whole, according to how healthy it is considered to be overall.

Once decided upon, the idea is that the traffic light system would be adopted as a standard across the food and drink industry so as to avoid confusion between different systems in different supermarkets and between different manufacturers.

It is not certain exactly when, or indeed if, this system will actually be adopted, but it is currently under research and the FSA certainly aim for it eventually to be put into use.

Why does it matter?

Maybe you are wondering what all the fuss is about over nutrients. So what if you have 'a lot' of sugar, or not much fibre? What exactly is the problem with having more than the day's GDA of fat? What's the problem with 'too much' of this or 'too little' of that?

Too much sugar

As you will have seen in Table 3 above, sugar in products comes in many forms. It is recommended that women of normal body weight, eating around 2,000 calories a day, have no more than 50g of sugar a day. Men eating 2,500 calories should stick to no more than 62g a day. None of these sugars supplies anything other than energy, which means that they are, in nutrition-speak, 'empty calories'. In other words, when added to foods and drinks they do not bring with them any useful vitamins or minerals, just energy.

And having sugary foods and drinks between meals, at times when you cannot brush your teeth, provides an ideal environment in your mouth for the growth of decay-causing bacteria. Steering away from sugary snacks and drinks between meals is a good idea if you want to look after your teeth.

Too much fat

Just one tablespoon of fat (15g), such as butter or margarine, gives us 111 calories worth of energy, once digested and absorbed. Because it is such a concentrated source of energy, it is easy to go overboard and clock up the calories when tucking away foods and drinks rich in fat.

That is one of the reasons why the guideline daily amounts suggest 70g a day for women and 95g for men as a maximum intake. For people wanting to lose weight, fat intake needs to be reduced along with the total amount of calories.

How much is too much fat?

People who want to reduce their calories should also look at reducing the total grams of fat they eat. Take a look at Table 4 below to get an idea of the levels of fat you should aim for when cutting back on calories.

Table 4

Total Calories Per Day	Total Fat Grams Per Day
1200	40g
1400	45g
1600	55g

Too much saturated fat

After eating foods and drinks containing saturated fats, the levels of LDL cholesterol rise in our blood. Raised LDL cholesterol increases the risk of this cholesterol sticking to blood vessel walls and causing blockages to the blood flow, which could trigger a heart attack or stroke.

When we eat polyunsaturated fats, for instance those found in sunflower oil, nuts and seeds, they seem to help to slightly lower the amount of LDL cholesterol in the blood. Mono-unsaturated fats, found for example in olive oil, on the other hand, tend to have a neutral effect on it.

Too little fibre

As I have mentioned, fibre comes in two forms. One type, which is found in apples and pears and foods like oats, is known as soluble fibre. This is because if you put it in water it forms a gel. When you eat foods rich in soluble fibre, the gel that forms in your digestive system has several benefits. It helps to make you feel full and also seems to help lower the cholesterol circulating in your blood. Eating lots of food rich in soluble fibre means you get these really useful benefits.

The other type, insoluble fibre, is found in foods like wholemeal bread, whole-grain breakfast cereals and brown rice. It is the husky, fibrous type that we cannot digest and it moves through our upper intestine and on into the colon. It gives our digestive system something to really get hold of and because it absorbs water, it bulks up our stools so that they pass easily through and reduce the risk of constipation.

By speeding the movement of stools through the colon it seems that this 'fibrous' fibre also helps to remove potential toxins and cancer-causing substances from the colon. Not having enough insoluble fibre may increase the risk of bowel problems like constipation or even cancer.

Adults in the UK eat around 12g of total fibre a day, which means that we need to up our intakes of vegetables, fruits and whole-grain foods if we are to reach the target of 18g a day for a healthy balanced diet.

Too much sodium or salt?

At the moment, we are packing away around 9g of salt a day – that is 3.6g of sodium. It is recommended that as adults we do not actually have more than 6g a day (or 2.5g sodium). Children's salt intake should be graded according to their age (see Table 5 for some salt intake guidelines).

Table 5 Salt intake guidelines

Age of child	Salt per day	Sodium per day	Equivalent teaspoons of salt per day
Up to 6 months	1g	0.4g	1/5
7–12 months	1g	0.4g	1/5
1–3 years	2g	0.8g	2/5
4–6 years	3g	1.2g	3/5
7–10 years	5g	2g	1

In most people, high salt intakes raise blood pressure, which in turn increases the likelihood of having a heart attack and stroke. A salt-rich diet also tends to encourage our bodies to hang on to excess body fluids. By reducing our salt intake to less than 3g a day (1.2g sodium), it has been suggested that we could lose one and a half litres of fluid, which amounts to 3lb in body weight. High intakes of salt have also been linked to an increased risk of developing the bone-thinning disease, osteoporosis.

And finally ...

 The nutrition label should help you to understand what contribution a food or drink is making to your diet nutritionally. It is up to the manufacturer whether or not they supply this information.

 If nutrition information is provided, the very least that must be present is 'The Big 4', which covers the energy in kJ and cal plus grams of protein, carbohydrate and fat.

 It is preferable for manufacturers to also supply details of 'The Big 4 plus Little 4', which includes the amount of carbohydrate that comes from sugar, the amount of fat that is saturated, plus the amount of fibre and salt a food supplies.

 It is helpful if labels supply nutritional information per serving and give guideline daily amounts. If these do not appear on the pack, you can check out the guidelines supplied in this chapter and take them with you when shopping.

You can do the same with the 'at a glance' guide (Table 3) to see when levels of a nutrient are considered to be high, medium or low.

If you use the information in this chapter you can really get to the bottom of nutrition labelling. It will help you make sense of, and put into perspective, the next chapter on Nutrition Claims and ensure you understand them for what they are.

3

Nutrition Claims

'Low Fat', 'High Fibre', 'Reduced Sugar'. We are so used to seeing these kinds of things splashed across our food labels these days that it is hard to imagine that even 25 years ago they were almost unheard of.

Most of us know which foods are naturally low in fat – vegetables and fruit, for example – and which foods are high in fibre, such as wholemeal bread. However, these days there are so many processed foods and drinks on our shelves that at first glance it is hard to know into which of these categories many of them fit.

For this reason, flashes on labels that tell us a food is 'Low in Salt' or 'High in Polyunsaturated Fats' can, in theory, be quite helpful when deciding what to put in our shopping baskets. However, as with all labelling, sometimes things are not quite as straightforward as they may seem. For a start, there is the distinction between absolute and relative nutrition claims.

Absolute and relative nutrition claims

■ Absolute claims are a statement of fact, such as '5g of Fat Per Serving'.

■ Relative claims provide nutritional comparisons with other foods, such as '25% Less Salt'.

Potential problems with nutrition claims

On the one hand, manufacturers cannot splash around nutrition claims on their foods and drinks if they are wildly untrue. To do so they would risk being hauled up in front of a judge and made to withdraw the product, scrap the packaging and start again from scratch.

On the other hand, with a few exceptions, at the present time there are no precise legal definitions regarding the exact levels of nutrients a product must contain in order for it to be allowed to use a claim like 'Low Fat'.

There are, however, voluntary guidelines. To be fair, most manufacturers do stick to these and we will have to make do until EU member states agree laws applicable across the whole of Europe. The big supermarkets and multinational food producers tend to go with them because, frankly, it is not worth the hassle to flaunt them.

Guidelines for nutrition claims

The Food Standards Agency have come up with these sensible guidelines for manufacturers to stick to regarding levels of nutrients and the claims that can be made about them:

Fat*

'Low Fat' – this means no more than 3g of fat per 100g or 100ml. Found, for example, on cottage cheese.

'Fat Free' – less than 0.15g of fat per 100g or 100ml. Found on some yoghurts.

'Low in Saturated Fat' – less than 1.5g of saturated fat per 100g and not more than 10 per cent of a food or drink's total calories. Found on vegetarian pate.

'Saturated-Fat Free' – less than 0.1g of saturated fat per 100g or 100ml.

Sugar

'Low Sugar' – this means less than 5g of sugar per 100g or 100ml. Found on, for example, some orange squash drinks.

'No Added Sugar' – no sugars, or foods composed mainly of sugars, added to the food or to any of its ingredients. Found on freshly squeezed orange juice.

These figures apply to all foods and drinks except margarine and spreads. They have their own set of rules which I discuss later.

'Sugar Free' – less than 0.2g of sugar per 100g or 100ml. Found on diet fizzy drinks.

Salt and sodium

'Low Sodium' – less than 40mg of sodium per 100g or 100ml of the food or drink. Found on, for example, some packs of muesli.

'No Added Salt' – no salt or sodium has been added to the food or any of its ingredients while it was made. Found on shredded wheat-style cereals and some rice cakes.

'Sodium/Salt Free' – less than 5mg sodium per 100g or 100ml of the food or drink.

Fibre

'A Source of Fibre' – the food must supply either 3g of fibre per 100g or 100ml, or at least 3g in the amount of food that you are likely to eat in an average day. Found on canned peas.

'Increased Fibre' – contains 25 per cent more fibre than a similar food for which no claims are made for fibre, or more than 3g per 100g or 100ml in the amount of food likely to be eaten in one day.

'% Fat Free' claims

In the past, you may have seen lots of products on the shelves that made a big song and dance about the fact that they were, for instance, '90% Fat Free' or '85% Fat Free'. Biscuits, cakes and crisps have, in the past, brandished these claims. But you may also have noticed that the number of them around is not as high these days.

This is because the voluntary guidelines for nutrition labelling recommend that they should no longer be used and most manufacturers are falling into step over this issue. This is a good thing. Why? Because '% Fat Free' labels can be really misleading. Surveys have revealed that when shoppers were shown a pack that claims to be '90% Fat Free' they believed the food to be lower in fat than another which said 'Low Fat'. But take a look at the facts here. '90% Fat Free' means that the food is still 10 per cent fat – that is 10g of fat per 100g. Yet the 'Low Fat' food might have had just 3 per cent fat – that is 3g of fat per 100g.

'90% Fat Free' shepherd's pie

You can get a feel of just how wonky the message of '% Fat Free' claims can really be when you look at an example of a ready-made meal. Let's use a Shepherd's Pie as an example.

If the Shepherd's Pie contained 10g of fat per 100g it could be described as being '90% Fat Free'. Yet, if you were to eat a 350g average serving of this ready-made Shepherd's Pie, you would be eating 35g of fat. For a woman, that is half of the 70g of fat she is aiming for in the day.

When '% Fat Free' claims are OK

The exception to manufacturers being advised against using '% Fat Free' claims is when a food contains less than 3g of fat, which means that it is genuinely low in fat. This means that it is reasonable for a manufacturer to flash up the fact that their product, such as a low-fat cracker with 3g of fat per 100g, is '97% Fat Free'.

Does 'Low Fat' mean low calories?

Sometimes, but not necessarily. Often calories in low-fat cakes and biscuits are not as low as you might imagine. When you take the fat out of milk to turn it from whole milk to skimmed milk, you just take the fat out, reducing it from 23g per pint to less than 1g per pint, and bringing the calories down from 385 per pint to 193. The only physical effect on the end product of removing the fat is that its consistency is thinner.

However, when you reduce the fat in a cake recipe you lose a lot of the cake's physical bulk, which must be replaced with another ingredient. This is usually sugar. A lot of sugar! A low-fat cake may then have quite similar calories to the standard version, as you can see from Table 6.

Table 6

	Grams of Fat	Calories
Whole milk per pint	23	385
Skimmed milk	0.6	193
Standard carrot cake per slice	5.0	98
Low-fat carrot cake	0.5	81

'Reduced' fat, sugar or salt

For a food or drink to claim that it has a 'reduced' amount of any nutrient, then the manufacturers should make sure that it has 25 per cent less of it than the original standard product. This means that you have to be a little circumspect when you spot 'reduced' labels, because for them to make sense you have to know how much of the nutrient would have appeared in the original. A 'reduced fat taramasalata', for instance, may have 25 per cent less fat than the standard taramasalata, but it still has 25g of fat per 100g. Reducing its fat by 25 per cent, while being a good thing, does not miraculously make it low in overall fat.

'Light' and 'Lite' claims

At the moment there are no laws covering the use of 'Light' and 'Lite' on packs. They are words that could be used to describe the texture of a food, or they could be used to imply that a food or drink has fewer calories or less fat than similar products. Because these claims can be a bit on the fuzzy side, manufacturers are asked to follow the suggested voluntary practice of using them only if their products comply with the principles covering 'reduced' claims, and therefore should only pop them on their labels if the products contain 25 per cent less fat, sugar or salt than their original counterparts.

'Virtually fat free'

This nutrition claim is in a real no-man's land. There are no voluntary guidelines for its use and no legal definitions. That said, it is used a lot on foods like yoghurts, and you can be pretty sure that if it does appear, then your food or drink is hardly supplying any fat.

Claims governed by law

While the nutrition claims above rely on manufacturers playing the role of good guys, there are some claims that are legally set in stone. The manufacturers can be liable for prosecution if they break the rules for these ones.

Energy

'Reduced Calorie'

A food and drink cannot say on its label that it is 'Reduced Calorie' unless it supplies no more than 75 per cent of a similar standard food. For example, a 'Reduced Calorie' orange squash.

'Low Calorie'

For a food or drink to claim to be 'Low Calorie' it must have fewer than 40 calories per normal serving size – that is equivalent to 167 kJ per 100g, or per 100ml. A 'Low Calorie' hot chocolate drink is a good example of this – one individual serving sachet of a typical low calorie chocolate drink, supplying 39 calories, would qualify for this claim.

Protein

Some foods and drinks, especially those designed for sports people or for helping people to convalesce, like to make a point that they are particularly good suppliers of protein.

The word protein *is flashed up on the label*
To even mention the word *protein* on the label the food must supply at least 12g of protein in a day's reasonable intake of the food.

'A source of protein'
For a product to actually claim to be a 'Source of Protein' it must supply more than 12 per cent of its total calories from protein.

'A rich or excellent source of protein'
For a product to go one step further and to state that it is a 'Rich' or 'Excellent Source' of protein, it must have more than 20 per cent protein; in other words, a fifth of calories must come from the protein it contains.

(Have another look at Chapter 2 if you want to get a feel for how much protein you need each day and why it is a crucial part of our diet.)

Cholesterol
This is an interesting one. The food laws say that to state a food has 'low cholesterol', it must have less than 5mg of cholesterol per 100g. To put this in perspective, eggs contain 231mg of cholesterol per egg, while a rye crispbread contains none.

In spite of this being the law, manufacturers are discouraged from drawing our attention to cholesterol levels because it is not the cholesterol in our foods that tends to lead to raised cholesterol in our blood. It is the level of saturated fats that we eat in things like fatty meat products, such as sausages and meat pies, and in cakes, biscuits and cream that raises blood cholesterol.

Vitamins and Minerals

Everything from breakfast cereals and 'morning' bars to fruit smoothies and even mineral water now show off about the vitamins and minerals they supply us with. But when it comes to vitamins and minerals manufacturers do have to be careful because, by law, there are certain levels of these that their products must supply to qualify for a claim.

'A source of vitamin C'

To be able to claim on a label that, for example, an orange juice is a 'Source of Vitamin C', it must provide a sixth of the recommended daily amount (RDA) of this vitamin. Since the RDA for vitamin C is 60mg, this means that it must provide 10mg in a serving before it can make this claim.

'A rich source of vitamin C'

For a product to boast that it is a 'Rich Source' it must supply half of the RDA. So the fruit drink would have to provide 30mg of vitamin C per serving.

'Contains vitamin C'

To even be able to mention the fact that it contains vitamin C, let alone say that it is a 'Source' or a 'Rich Source', the juice has to supply a minimum of 15 per cent of the RDA, which for vitamin C would be 9mg.

Every vitamin and mineral have a different RDA (see Table 7) and so the levels at which each can justify being mentioned on a pack are different for each one.

'High in vitamins or minerals'

Currently, the voluntary advice regarding claims that a food or drink is 'High' in certain vitamins and minerals is that this should only be used when the product supplies at least twice the amount allowed for 'A Source of' claim – in other words, a third of the RDA.

'Reduced-Fat', 'Low-Fat' and 'Extra Low-Fat' spreads

When it comes to 'Reduced-Fat', 'Low-Fat' or 'Extra Low-Fat' claims on spreads, forget the rules that apply to other foods. They have their own set and these rules are legally enforceable.

- To be 'Low Fat', a spread must contain less than 40g of fat per 100g.
- To be 'Very Low Fat', it must contain no more than 20–30g.

As you can see, these cut-off points mean that the spreads, whether low or very low fat, are still high in total fat. It is just that they are low and very low compared to the 82g of fat per 100g in butter and margarine.

Table 7 RDAs for vitamins and minerals

Vitamins	
Vitamin A	800µg
Vitamin B1 (thiamin)	1.4mg
Vitamin B2 (riboflavin)	1.6mg
Niacin	18.0mg
Vitamin B6	2.0µg
Vitamin B12	1.0µg
Biotin	0.15mg
Pantothenic acid	6.0mg
Vitamin C	60mg
Vitamin D	5.0µg
Vitamin E	10mg
Minerals	
Calcium	800mg
Iodine	150µg
Iron	14mg
Phosphorus	800mg
Magnesium	300mg
Zinc	15mg

µg = micrograms
mg = milligrams

FREQUENTLY ASKED QUESTIONS

Q. *Why do some brands of 'Reduced-Fat' crisps contain more fat than standard versions of other crisps?*

A. The term 'Reduced-Fat' applies to the reduction compared to the same brand's full-fat version. If brand X has quite a bit more fat than brand Y, brand X's 'Reduced-Fat' version may still have more total fat than brand Y's original version. Always check the product's nutritional credentials per total serving before buying it if you are consciously cutting down on fat.

Q. *If a food claims to be 'Low Fat', can I assume it is healthy?*

A. Not necessarily. It could, for example, be low in fat, yet high in sugar. 'Low-Fat' and 'Reduced-Fat' cakes and biscuits are a classic example of this kind of pitfall, because when you lower the amount of fat you use in a recipe to make cakes and biscuits, you have to put something else in to replace it, otherwise there will not be sufficient bulk. Usually, when fat is reduced, it is sugar that is piled in to take its place. Which means that you can pat yourself on the back for choosing a low-fat cake while unwittingly be wading into a food that is jam-packed with sugar.

In the long run, this can be a problem if you are watching your weight because sometimes the massive amounts of sugar added to replace the fat bring the final calories up to pretty much the same as those in the original version. Bonkers, but true!

Q. *How can I make sense of 'Low-Fat' claims then?*

A. Do not rely on the fat claim. Take a look at how many calories you are getting per serving of the cake. At the end of the day, if you are watching your weight, it is the total number of calories you are eating each day that will make the difference on the weighing scales.

Q. *I always think, 'Oh great, because this food is low in fat, or reduced in fat, then I may as well have two!' I suppose this isn't very sensible, is it?*

A. It is another little trap into which it is human nature to fall. The idea that you are being 'good' because you are selecting a low-fat food can make it really tempting to have two instead of one. Do this and you would probably have been better off just having one of the standard version of the product.

Q. *What does it mean when a label says a food is 'Naturally Low in Sugar'?*

A. Some foods are naturally low in fat, salt or sugar. When this is the case, manufacturers should not make a big thing about it by putting flashes on the product saying 'Low Fat' or 'Low Sugar'. Instead, because they are just implicitly low, the advice is that the label should say:

'A Low-Fat Food'
'A Low-Saturates Food'
'A Low-Sugar Food'
'A Low-Salt (or Sodium) Food'
'A High-Fibre Food'

By using this kind of description it is hoped that the nutrient claim will not be misleading.

Q. *Many of the foods and drinks I see in the supermarkets say they have, for example, extra added calcium or minerals. Are these good ways to get the extra nutrients? Is, for example, the calcium added to calcium-enriched orange juice as good a way to get calcium as getting it from milk or other dairy products?*

A. In some cases, such as orange juices or soya milk that have added calcium, these can be really useful sources of this nutrient, especially for people who do not eat dairy foods like milk or yoghurt, which are traditionally good suppliers of calcium. However, I've seen 'Added Calcium' flashed across foods marketed for children's lunch boxes which are based on processed cheese. These products are rich in salt, contain quite a lot of additives and have questionable overall nutritional value. In such cases, the calcium claim is, in my view, a bit misleading.

And finally ...

When European laws eventually kick into action regarding nutrition labelling, hopefully the pitfalls will become fewer and further between. Until then, remember that it is possible for a manufacturer to draw your attention to his product being low in one nutrient when it is screamingly high in another. Always remember:

Don't be seduced by first impressions.

Don't take every claim you see at face value.

Flip the product over and take a look at the nutrient box.

If in doubt, leave it on the shelf.

Only add it to your trolley when you are completely satisfied that a product is what it seems.

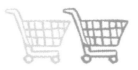

4

Health Claims

The idea that certain foods and drinks are 'good' for us is not new. We know that fish is 'good' for our brains and that carrots help us to see in the dark – this knowledge has been passed down through word of mouth over the centuries, and scientists today are proving such folklore to be true.

These days, food labels are trying to do a similar job by informing us of their benefits through the health claims they make on their food labels and packaging.

The facts about health claims

■ Like nutrition claims, there are no special laws in place at the moment that govern health claims, but there are voluntary guidelines that manufacturers should follow so that claims on a pack are not misleading or false.

■ However, it is illegal to say that a food directly cures, treats or prevents an illness, since this would make the food or drink a medicine, which would mean it would need to be prescribed by your doctor.

These are the kind of health claims that can be made for a food or drink:

- that they can help maintain good health in general;
- that they can help maintain the health of a specific part of the body, like the heart or digestive system;
- that they can help to reduce the risk factor of a disease, like reducing cholesterol, if it is also explained that they do so as part of a healthy lifestyle.

These health claims can be for:

- the food itself – for example, a 100 per cent whole-grain breakfast cereal;

- a nutrient in the food – for example, the mineral calcium in mineral water;
- an added ingredient – for example, added 'good' (probiotic) bacteria to a yoghurt.

The guidelines

As they stand, the guidelines covering health claims apply to any words, trademarks, brand names, pictures on the packaging or symbols on the label, as well as any little extra collars around bottle tops, any special peel-off labels attached to, or special notices on, the packs.

As well as helping to guide the makers of foods and drinks to make honest health claims on their labels, the guidelines should also be followed by the people who are paid to advertise and promote the products.

If you see a food carrying a claim saying, for example, that it can 'Treat or Cure Arthritis', then you can complain to your local council's Trading Standards Officer, who will investigate and hopefully have it removed from sale.

Other important points about health claims

- It is really important that when a product carries a health claim, the label tells you the serving size you need in order to reap the health benefit.
- If there are certain people at whom the product is aimed – pregnant women, older people, or children, for example – the label should tell you so.

- If there are any people who should avoid the food, the label needs to make this clear.
- If a high intake of the food could be harmful, the label must tell you and give a safe maximum intake.

Health claims you may see on labels

For your digestive system

'Maintains bowel regularity, which can help to ensure a healthy digestion and bowel.'

'Is beneficial to the health of the stomach and digestive system.'

A yoghurt with added 'good' (probiotic) bacteria, for example, may say on its label: 'Can help keep your digestive system in balance.'

For your heart and circulation

'Contributes to a healthy metabolism and blood circulation, which keeps the heart and blood vessels clear and healthy.'

'Helps maintain normal blood flow to the brain, which is particularly important in old age.'

'Helps maintain normal cholesterol levels. Healthy cholesterol levels are known to play a part in maintaining a healthy heart.'

For example, a margarine that is rich in polyunsaturated fats may say on its label: 'Helping to keep your heart healthy. With sunflower goodness and essential polyunsaturates, this helps as part of a healthy diet.'

A 100 per cent whole-grain breakfast cereal may say: 'People with healthy hearts tend to eat more whole-grain foods as part of a low-fat diet and healthy lifestyle.'

For your immune system
'Provides nutrients that are needed to ensure a healthy immune system for convalescents'.

For your blood pressure
'Good for your blood pressure, which helps to maintain a healthy heart and normal blood flow to the body'.

Claim now, check later

At the moment, the makers of foods and drinks can add a health claim to the food or drink before they put it on the shelves of our supermarkets. Consumer groups would like to see a law passed that would mean manufacturers would have to get 'prior approval'. In other words, they would have to go through a Health Claims Body and say, 'Look, this is the claim I'd like to make, here's the evidence, what do you think?' If the answer were 'yes', then fair enough. If the product does what the makers say it does, then the claim would be approved and added to the pack.

It would be good, too, if the law said that health claims could only be allowed on foods that are all-round 'good guys' on the nutritional front. This would stop a food like a wholemeal banana cake containing lots of fibre, for example, telling us it was good for our digestion if was also packed with sugar and salt that are good neither for our teeth nor our blood pressure.

Specific health claims that get the 'thumbs up'

At the moment, although the general claims mentioned above are allowed to be used on foods and drinks, there are some specific health claims that have been given a particular 'thumbs up' by the people who created the voluntary guidelines.

Called the Joint Health Claims Initiative, this body has only given permission for a few of these claims to be used on a select few foods, after plenty of consideration of the scientific facts. Specific claims are only allowed when a food or drink (or a nutrient or added ingredient that it contains) really has been able to prove through plenty of good research that it is able to make a significant contribution to our health. (*Check out Chapter 12 on Functional Food to find out more.*)

Specific health claims that have been given approval

Soya protein and blood cholesterol

- Makers of foods rich in soya protein could put the following claim on their packs of, for example, soya milk and tofu (soya-bean curd): 'The inclusion of at least 25g of soya protein per day, as part of a diet low in saturated fat, can help reduce blood cholesterol.'

- Any food, like soya milk for instance, that carries the claim must be able to provide at least 6.25g of soya protein per serving, and must tell you what proportion of your optimum 25g total it supplies.

- For example, soya milk may carry the health claim saying: 'At least 25g of soya protein a day, as part of a diet low in saturated fats, can help reduce cholesterol in the blood. Contains 9.3g of soya protein per serving. One serving is 250ml.'
- Manufacturers are not allowed to use the claim if the food is not low in saturated fat, even though it contains the right amount of soya protein.

Whole-grain foods and a healthy heart

- Certain claims about eating whole-grain foods can be made in relation to heart health. For example: 'People with a healthy heart tend to eat more whole-grain foods as part of a healthy lifestyle.'
- Makers of porridge, for example, can say on their label: 'Porridge oats are rich in soluble fibre which, when eaten as part of a low-fat diet, can help maintain a healthy heart. Each serving contains 30 per cent of the 3g of soluble oat fibre required per day to help maintain a healthy heart. One serving is 39g.'

Reducing saturated fats and blood cholesterol

- A claim can be made on foods that help to reduce saturated fat and blood cholesterol. The claim allowed is: 'Decreasing dietary saturates (saturated fat) can help lower blood cholesterol.'
- This claim cannot be used on the labels of foods targeted at children who are less than two years of age.

- On a polyunsaturated margarine you may therefore find: 'Helping to keep your heart healthy. Using this margarine as part of a healthy diet can help lower cholesterol.'

Reducing cholesterol using plant stanol and plant sterol esters

- Plant stanols and plant sterol esters naturally exist in some plants and are now added to certain brands of margarine and yoghurt. They have been shown to help lower cholesterol in the blood by latching onto cholesterol in the digestive system and carrying it out of the body in the stools. They can now be added to certain foods.
- Specific claims can be made for these ingredients: 'This spread contains a unique ingredient called plant stanol ester, which can actually help to lower cholesterol as part of a healthy diet.'
- A spread containing plant stanol esters may say: 'Proven to reduce cholesterol as part of a healthy diet. Recommended serving: two-to-three servings a day. One serving is 12g of spread.'

FREQUENTLY ASKED QUESTIONS

Q. *Are supermarket 'Healthy Eating' ranges healthier and better than buying the usual version?*

A. Not always. Surveys by consumer groups have discovered that often when fat levels are lowered in foods like cakes and biscuits, sugar and salt levels go up. In ready-made meals the fat may be reduced by simply cutting back on the amount of meat in the product and adding fillers and even sugar to bulk it back up. Until labelling laws are put in place to ensure that foods purporting to be healthy really are healthy from a holistic point of view, you do need to read the label to check exactly what you are getting in 'Healthy Eating' ranges.

The same goes for children's 'Healthy Eating' ranges. Many have cut back on additives, but do take an all-round look at them to check what you are getting.

Q. *A tin of spaghetti hoops I bought had a logo on it claiming that it counted as a serving of vegetables. How can this be the case?*

A. The manufacturers say that the tomato sauce in which the spaghetti hoops come counts as a serving of vegetables. Personally, I think this is bonkers! The tomato sauce may contain puréed tomatoes but it is also rich in salt and sugar. If you were to make a quick tomato sauce at home and pour it over a bowl of cooked pasta you would benefit from the skins and seeds of the tomatoes, which supply extra protective nutrients, fibre and supernutrients, minus the sugar and with far less salt.

And finally ...

Even though there is a voluntary set of guidelines that food and drink producers should follow so that they do not make false health claims about their products, some do slip through the net. Ensure that you are not caught out by following these golden rules:

If a claim sounds too good to be true – perhaps a drink claims to boost your sex life – the chances are it *is* too good to be true. Use your judgement and common sense and do not be taken in by the hype. If you think the claim is unsound, report it to the Trading Standards Officer of your local council.

If a food that you would normally think of as being 'unhealthy', such as a chocolate bar, carries a health claim such as 'rich in antioxidants that can help maintain a healthy heart', then consider the bigger picture. True, it may well contain antioxidants, but it is also rich in fat, sugar and calories. In the case of chocolate bars with health claims, forget them. Have an apple instead, which is naturally rich in antioxidants and low in calories too.

If the name of a product implies a health claim, be really sceptical. For instance, a drink called 'Morning-After Detox' implies that it may help to cure a hangover. In fact, there is very little that you can do to cure a hangover other than take some paracetamol, drink lots of water and wait until your body has naturally restored itself to a state of balance.

A picture speaks a thousand words. If a picture on the label implies that a food or drink will improve your health – for example, maybe it has a picture of a heart that suggests it is good for your heart – do not just take the suggestion at face value. Check out the ingredients label and, if there is one, the nutrition label too, to see what it really contains.

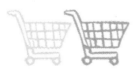

5

Glycaemic index

The glycaemic index

Another symbol that you will find increasing popping up on certain food and drink labels is the 'GI' symbol. GI stands for glycaemic index. Only products that contain carbohydrate will carry such information because the GI is a means of classifying the speed with which carbohydrate is broken down during digestion and how quickly or slowly and how profoundly it affects sugar levels in our blood after eating it.

The most obvious carbohydrate foods and drinks that usually spring to mind are bread and potatoes, rice and pasta. But carbohydrates come in many forms and not just as these typical and well-known 'starchy' types. Fruit, some vegetables and everything from honey and sugar to foods containing these ingredients, such as cakes, biscuits and sweets, are all carbohydrates as are drinks such as juices and squash.

While they may start life in very different forms, all with unique appearances, textures and tastes, once chewed, swallowed and digested, all are ultimately broken down into glucose (also known as 'blood sugar') in the blood.

It may seem hard to imagine a piece of French stick and a jelly bean both meeting the same metabolic fate, but this dismantling of carbohydrate from different starting points down into glucose is a crucial step to survival because glucose is the energy currency of all cells, powering every thing from activity in our brains to the pumping of our hearts.

The GI value of a carbohydrate is worked out by comparing the speed at which it is digested and its subsequent effects on glucose levels in the blood, with the effects of eating pure glucose.

Glucose is given a score of 100 against which other carbohydrates are measured. A food with a GI index under 55 is considered to have a low GI. Scientists have discovered that when we base our meals and snacks around low-GI carbohydrates, they tend to keep us feeling fuller for longer, which is useful when losing weight. They also appear to offer protection against heart disease and help people with diabetes to control their blood sugar levels.

Foods with a medium GI of 55–70 raise blood sugar levels more rapidly than low-GI foods. When following a low-GI eating plan it is wise to eat these only in moderation.

Carbohydrate foods and drinks with a high GI of over 70 should be avoided most of the time when following a low-GI plan. They raise sugar levels in the blood rapidly. The problem with such fast rises is that in turn our body responds by pumping out a lot of the hormone insulin from the pancreas to bring blood glucose levels back down. Excessive amounts of insulin cart the excess glucose out of the blood, from where it is converted into and stored as fat. Meantime we are left feeling hungry soon after.

While GI labelling may help to guide us to low-GI foods, this system is not widely in use as yet. It is therefore useful to get an understanding of the various factors that influence the GI value of foods and drinks so that you are able to make your own judgements as to whether a food is likely to be high, medium or low GI when out and about shopping.

It is also important to understand why some medium-GI foods that appear to be fine to eat in moderation, actually would be detrimental to a weight loss plan. I always believe that forewarned is forearmed when it comes to unravelling labelling in the supermarkets.

Factors that influence GI values of carbohydrate foods and drinks

What makes a carbohydrate low, high or indeed medium GI is in some cases fairly logical.

Processing

The more processed a carbohydrate, the higher its GI tends to be. A breakfast cereal like cornflakes, for instance, which has undergone heat treatment and had sugar added has a high GI compared to porridge oats, which have undergone no processing except rolling.

The cornflakes have in a sense already been partially 'digested' during the processing, making it easier for our enzymes to then complete the job. Because the cornflakes take little digestion, it means that they raise glucose in our blood extremely quickly and to quite high levels.

Types of fibre

The type of fibre a carbohydrate contains also affects its GI value. Those containing a type of fibre that becomes 'jelly-like' when it is mixed with fluid in the stomach, like the pectin in pears or apples for example, will slow digestion of their starchy part and lower their GI. Oats also contain this viscous type of fibre. It is quite easy to imagine a gluey mass in the stomach and intestine holding up the digestive process.

It is also simple to understand how the fibrous outer skins which coat pulses like baked beans and, say, red kidney beans act as a physical barrier during digestion, slowing down the rate at which digestive enzymes can get in to the middle part of the bean and begin its breakdown.

This is true too of breads containing whole grains like multigrain bread. With wholemeal bread, during milling, wheat grains have their fibrous coat removed from the starchy grain. The fibre is separately ground up and then added back. Although the resulting flour and bread is high in fibre, the starchy grains are free and easily accessed by digestive enzymes and so rapidly broken into glucose.

With multigrain bread enzymes have to break their way through the outer husk of the whole wheat grains. This explains why wholemeal bread has a higher GI than multigrain bread.

Sometimes the GI of a food is not quite so logical and needs a more in-depth understanding.

Type of starch

It all gets a bit more complex when it comes to the different types of starch a carbohydrate contains. One type of starch is called amylose and another, amylopectin. In amylose the glucose molecules are lined up tightly together and form close-knit clumps that are a struggle for digestive enzymes to break into. Basmati rice, for instance, has lots of amylose starch.

In amylopectin starch the glucose molecules are branching out all over the place giving lots of access to the enzymes. Standard white rice is a good example of an amylopectin-rich carbohydrate.

The difference in the types of starches in these foods explains why basmati rice is a medium-GI food and white rice is high.

Cooking

Cooking can increase the GI of a food. When a potato is baked for a long period, the starch granules inside become very fluffy and digestive enzymes have easy access to break them down very rapidly, which causes quick rises in blood sugar and makes them a high-GI food.

New boiled potatoes, however, have starch granules which

are still quite tightly packed together after boiling, a fact that makes them a medium-GI food.

As you can see, when following a low-GI diet you need to be prepared to ditch your previous preconceptions of what is a 'healthy carbohydrate' and what is not. For instance, baked potatoes have traditionally been perceived as being a great diet food. They are after all low in fat. The problem is that they are broken down into glucose in a just a flash, faster in fact than jelly beans.

I am not, however, suggesting that jelly beans make for a more slimming lunch than baked potatoes. Baked potatoes have lots of good points such as fibre in their skins for a healthy colon. But new potatoes boiled in their skin would make a better GI choice.

Acid

Vinegar and lemon juice when eaten with a meal significantly lower the GI value of a meal. A tablespoon of vinaigrette dressing can reduce the blood sugar levels by as much as 30 per cent. This seems to be because acid helps to slow the rate at which the stomach empties itself of food, which in turn means that all nutrients, including carbohydrates are digested more slowly. Research carried out at the University of Sydney has shown that wine vinegar and lemon juice have the greatest effect on lowering the GI value of a meal (balsamic vinegar is also useful).

This understanding of acid reducing GI helps to explain why sourdough bread is more slowly digested than standard white bread. Its slightly acidic nature is due to the lactic acid and propionic acid it contains, which are produced during fermentation.

Adding sugar

The presence of added sugar affects the GI of food. Adding sugar to canned fruit will push its GI from low when canned in fruit juice to medium when canned in sugar. A diet yoghurt sweetened with an artificial intense sweetener or a plain yoghurt is low GI compared with one with added sugar, which is medium.

Putting theory into practice

To make life simple you need to be aware of and accept these points. It does seem bizarre that bagels are high GI, whereas pitta breads are low. But if you do not believe the scientists, do a test on yourself. Eat one of each on its own and monitor how long it is before you next feel peckish. I guarantee you will be hankering after the biscuit tin much sooner after the bagel compared to the low-GI pitta.

This is where GI labelling may be useful. You may not have known that pitta is low GI, but with a 'Low GI' symbol on the pack, you will be able to make an informed low-GI choice in the bakery section when shopping.

Low GI is not always 'healthy'

As with most things in life, there are of course some exceptions to the rules. Not all foods and drinks boasting a 'low' or 'medium' GI symbol should be in your shopping trolley if you are trying to lose or maintain your weight. This is when you need to be aware that just because a food or drink has a low or medium GI, it is not necessarily low in calories.

Chocolate

Chocolate could in theory carry a 'Low GI' symbol and soon some brands probably will use this as a way of marketing it to customers. The reason that chocolate has a GI of just 49 is because the absorption of sugar in chocolate (56g per 100g bar) is slowed down by the presence of a large amount of fat (31g of fat per 100g bar). The overall effect is that chocolate does not affect blood sugar drastically but it can, because it contains 520 calories per 100g bar, certainly hinder weight loss.

Popcorn

Popcorn has a GI of 55. Like corn, popcorn just scrapes in as a low-GI food and could carry a 'Low GI' label. The healthiest popcorn is prepared at home from bagged popping corn in an air popper. But even then you should still go very steady. Standard salted popcorn you buy, for instance, at the cinema is popped in oil and has 444 calories and 32g of fat for just a small 100g box and will wreck your weight loss plans. Obviously sweet popcorn is out. It has a higher GI and is loaded with a similar number of calories to the salted version.

Crisps

Crisps have a GI of 54 and again could carry a 'Low GI' symbol on pack. This is not because they have overnight turned into a 'health' food. The fat used to fry the crisps brings the GI of potatoes down from being in the 80s, and thus a high-GI food, to 54, making it a low-GI food. The oil, however, means that the crisps are rich in calories – a 50g bag provides 215 calories.

Sausages

Sausages have a GI of 28. Although we think of sausages as being a meat and therefore not having a GI, they contain lots of cereals and so do appear on GI tables. The fact that they appear in the low-GI column may lead to confusion and to people thinking they are healthy. In fact reduced fat versions can be quite good choices when slimming; however, standard sausages contain a lot of fat and are not. It is the presence of both this fat and the protein in the meat in sausages that makes the GI number so low. Two pork sausages supply about 300 calories and 22g of fat.

Fish fingers

These have a GI of 38. They have a GI number because they are coated in breadcrumbs and because the GI is low, there is a temptation to think they are healthy. But when fried, four fish fingers supply 280 calories and 16g of fat. You are much better off with 150g of white fish for 150 calories and zero fat.

Chocolate-flavoured milk

This drink has a GI of just 34, which makes it seem as though you can slosh it down no bars held. But remember, a 500ml bottle of this milk supplies 325 calories and around 40g of sugar. The sugar absorption is slowed down by the fat in the milk, but the calories can pile on the pounds.

Apple muffins

With a GI of 44, muffins again are a wolf in sheep's clothing because the reality is that they can have a good 500 calories each. Home made versions can be healthier when little fat is used and sugar is replaced by fructose, but do not be fooled that commercially available apple muffins are a 'good thing' to be regularly tucking into.

Banana cake

The same goes for banana cake with a GI of 47. The fat in this cake along with the banana it contains will slow down the absorption of the added sugars. But remember that a slice can supply 350 calories, 14g of fat and 36g of sugar.

Sponge cake

With a GI of 46, sponge cake also seems innocent enough. Again go steady. Some 467 calories for a 100g slice is hardly good for the waistline.

Fruit juices

Most fruit juices such as orange, apple and grapefruit have a GI of 40. These are not harmful, but it is easy to go overboard on fruit juices. Stick to a 200ml serving and that's around 100 calories. Glug down a litre and you have drunk 500 of your daily calorie intake.

Ice cream

With a GI of 61, ice cream could carry a 'Medium GI' symbol because, like chocolate, its fat content slows down the absorption of its sugar. But the fact remains that two scoops of even the most standard, non-glam ice-cream provide 264 calories, 14g of fat and 7 teaspoons of sugar.

High GI is not always 'bad'

Although baked potatoes have a high GI, they are usually eaten as part of a meal. The same goes for white bread or a bagel. Protein and fat in a meal and foods with a good amount of soluble fibre like baked or red kidney beans counteract the high GI of these carbohydrates and help to lower the overall GI of the meal.

This means that a high-GI baked potato when eaten with a high-protein or low-GI filling like chilli con carne or baked beans or a high-GI bagel eaten with smoked salmon or topped with tuna and sweetcorn becomes, overall, a medium-GI meal.

Because some high-GI foods such as these are nutritious, it is good to find ways of toning down their GI status so that we can still enjoy them in our meals and snacks.

Losing weight when going low GI

Although the absolute backbone of low GI dieting revolves around selecting mostly low- and some medium-GI carbo-hydrates, while eschewing high-GI versions, it is also vital to choose sensibly from the other two food groups – protein and fats.

As far as protein foods are concerned this means sticking with chicken – without the skin and not fried chicken obviously, extra lean red meats and fish. Go for lower-fat versions of milk and dairy foods. Protein foods also include eggs, which are fine so long as you don't have a cholesterol problem, lean bacon and foods like Quorn and tofu. For fats then it is vital to go steady. Those you do choose should be the types that provide some useful essential fats and nutrients like olive oil, nuts and seeds.

Alcohol is always a mute point when shedding pounds. For maximum losses of two pounds a week it is hard to drink daily and succeed in achieving your goal. Once you have reached your target weight, there is no reason not to enjoy your favourite tipple because low GI is for life, not just a mad attempt to shed the annual January pounds.

Table 8 shows some examples of lower-GI foods versus higher-GI foods to help get you into the swing of things.

Table 8

LOWER GI	HIGHER GI
Breakfast cereals	
Porridge	Golden syrup flavoured micro-
Muesli (sugar free)	waveable porridge
Sultana Bran	Crunchy sugar-coated muesli
	Cornflakes
Breads	
Granary	White / wholemeal bread
Rye	Standard 'brown' bread
Sourdough bread	Ciabatta bread
Rice & cereals	
Basmati rice	Long grain rice
Wild rice	Brown rice
Pasta	Bagels
Vegetables	
Boiled new potatoes	Mashed potatoes
Sweet potatoes	Baked standard potatoes
Spinach, broccoli, mange tout	Parsnips
Fruit	
Fresh fruit salad in juice	Canned fruit salad in syrup
Medium ripe banana	Over-ripe banana
Canteloupe melon	Watermelon
Snacks	
Oatcakes	Custard creams
Plain popcorn	Toffee popcorn
Plain yoghurt	Fruit yoghurt with added sugar

Table 9 provides a more comprehensive list of foods with a GI of 55 or under. The lower the GI of the foods you choose, the better.

Table 9

Low fat popcorn	55
Fruit salad	55
Banana	55
Mango	55
Sweetcorn	55
Linseed rye bread	55
Oat bran	55
Semolina	55
Sweet potatoes	54
Buckwheat	54
Gram dhal	54
Oatmeal biscuits	54
Sultana bran	52
Kiwi	52
Kidney beans (canned)	52
Sultan Bran cereal	52
Yam	51
Chocolate	49
Bulghur (cooked)	48
Grapefruit juice	48
Peas	48
Boiled carrots	49

cont.

Fruit loaf (heavy)	47
Noodles	46
Orange juice	46
Grapes	46
Pineapple juice	46
Pinto beans	45
Oranges	44
Lentil soup	44
Muesli	43
Custard	43
Toasted muesli	43
Porridge	42
All Bran	42
Peaches	42
Lentil soup	42
Pumpernickel bread	41
Pasta	40
Apple juice	40
Rice noodles	40
Plums	39
Mung bean noodles	39
Ravioli	39
Apples	38
Pears	38
Haricot beans	38
Yoghurt (plain)	37
Chickpeas (boiled)	33

cont.

Table 9 (*cont.*)

Butter beans	31
Dried apricots	31
Black beans (boiled)	30
Lentils	28
Milk	27
Red kidney beans	27
Grapefruit	25
Pearl barley (boiled)	25
Fructose	23
Cherries	22
Rice bran	19
Soy beans	18
Black gram (boiled)	16
Peanuts	14

The foods listed in Table 10 have a high GI of 70 and above and are the ones that need to be replaced with low-GI foods.

Table 10

Glucose	100
Glutinous white rice	98
Boiled parsnips	97
French bread	95
Rice pasta	92
White rice	87

Corn flakes	84
Instant mash	83
Rice Krispies	82
Rice cakes	82
Puffed wheat	80
Jelly beans	80
Rich Tea biscuits	79
Canned lychee	79
Water biscuits	78
Co Co Pops	77
Brown rice	76
Waffles	76
French fries	75
Pumpkin	75
Cream crackers	74
Soda crackers	74
Bagel	72
Watermelon	72
Baked potatoes	72
Grapenuts	71
Millet	71
Tapioca	71
White bread	70

The foods listed in Table 11 have a medium GI (above 55 and under 70). The idea is to go steady on these and have lower-GI versions where you can.

Table 11

Ryvita	69
Crumpets	69
Bran flakes	68
Croissant	67
New potatoes	66
Pineapple	66
Cantaloupe melon	65
Sugar	65
Raisins	64
Muesli bars	61
Ice cream	61
Papaya	58
Honey	58
Pitta bread	57
Sultanas	56
Bananas	55
Sweetcorn	55
Crisps	54

Who is using GI labelling?

People living in Australia are already very familiar with GI labelling on their foods and drinks. Presently in the UK, the supermarket chain Tesco is at the forefront of GI labelling.

The supermarket is labelling products with low- and medium-GI symbols, although not surprisingly, products will not carry high-GI symbols. No supermarket wants to put its customers off buying its foods!

The Tesco labelling system has been made possible by scientists from Oxford Brookes University testing the GI rating of everyday foods to ensure accurate labelling. It is estimated that around one thousand foods and drinks in Tesco stores will eventually carry a GI symbol on their labels, including bread and pasta, ready meals and breakfast cereals.

Other manufacturers seem very likely to follow this new form of nutritional labelling. There is currently no specific law to which GI labelling must conform, although, as with all labelling on food, it must comply with basic labelling laws and be honest, legal and decent.

FREQUENTLY ASKED QUESTIONS

Q. *Can I eat as much as I like of low-GI foods and still lose weight?*

A. No. Low GI foods and drinks are simply digested more slowly than medium- and high-GI foods and tend to keep you feeling fuller for longer, which is why they help you to lose weight. If you over-ride your natural appetite and hunger signals and pile into huge bowls of muesli and loaves of pumpernickel bread you will gain, not lose, weight.

Q. *Will GI symbols appear on all brands of foods in all supermarkets?*

A. At the moment it is only one supermarket that has taken the initiative and a handful of manufacturers. Others may follow suit. In order to do so, however, they need to have each food individually tested by a reputable body to determine the GI value. This is a costly and lengthy process so the increase in GI labelling will probably be slower rather faster.

Q. *Is it safe to feed children low-GI foods?*

A. Yes. A low-GI diet is a healthy way of eating which is suitable for all the family. It is, after all, how we always used to eat and the basis on which culinary traditions such as Mediterranean and Asian diets have evolved over centuries.

And finally ...

 The GI index is a score of between 1 and 100, which ranks carbohydrate-containing foods and drinks according to their effect immediately after eating on levels of sugar in our blood.

 Those that are broken down rapidly and give a high rise in blood sugar are 'High GI' foods and drinks. Those that are broken down slowly and give a slow rise in blood sugar are 'Low GI'.

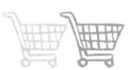 High-GI foods and drinks trigger a large rush of the hormone insulin to be released into the blood to restore blood sugar to normal levels. Research has led medical and nutritional experts to believe that high insulin levels encourage fat storage, discourage fat burning and leave us craving for more high-GI carbohydrates.

Low-GI foods on the other hand cause low insulin levels, which encourages fat burning, discourages fat storage and naturally curbs hunger, helping us to unhitch ourselves from constant cravings and to rely not on willpower to eat less, but on our exquisitely designed inner hunger signals to tell us when it is time to eat and when it is time to stop.

It is important to grasp, however, that not all high-GI foods are 'bad' and not all low-GI foods are 'good'.

It is a good idea to know the GI values of common foods so that you are not fooled by low- and medium-GI foods which are labelled as such in supermarkets but which are not necessarily 'healthy'.

6

Low Carbs

If there is one area of food labelling which is in a real state of disarray it is without doubt the labelling of a relatively new type of products – low-carbohydrate foods and drinks.

Fuelled by the recent obsession with high-protein dieting, which involves dramatically cutting the quantity and improving the type of carbohydrates eaten, the low-carbohydrate section in supermarkets and health food stores is steadily growing. From soup to jam, breakfast cereals to instant mashed potato, bread and chocolate, low-carbohydrate foods and drinks are becoming quite familiar.

If you are tempted to buy any of these foods, it is definitely worth getting to the bottom of the highly unique and, in my view, potentially confusing labelling used on these products.

As with glycaemic index (GI) labelling (see Chapter 5), low-carbohydrate labels do not have any special laws governing their use at present, and therefore have no legal definition. This means that as long as they are 'legal, decent and honest', they can continue in their confusing, merry way. In fact, I would take issue that many are not actually honest because they are so confusing, but that is another story. Right now it is important to get down to deciphering what low-carbohydrate eating is about and what the labels actually mean.

Why low carb?

Lots of people have been cutting carbohydrate in their diets in an effort to follow high-protein eating plans. The idea is to reduce, in the first two weeks of the diet, carbohydrate intakes right down from around 200–300g a day in the form of breakfast cereals, bread, pasta, rice, potatoes, fruit, sweets, cakes and biscuits to a meagre 20g a day, which comes from a small serving of vegetables or salad. By having so little carbohydrate, the body is forced to burn fat as fuel.

After the initial two-week period, high-protein diet followers are then allowed carbohydrate up to 60–100g a day. The types of carbohydrate eaten must be those that raise blood sugar levels slowly and gently give only small increases in the hormone insulin. In this sense this phase of the diet shares the same theory as the low-GI diet. The idea being that by keeping insulin levels down, more fat is burnt, and we feel fuller for longer.

With high-protein diets, however, the use of low-carbohydrate products is encouraged so as to keep the total amount of carbohydrate eaten below 100g a day.

How can you lower carbohydrate in high-carbohydrate foods?

Bread, bagels, pitta, crackers and crisps

In these kinds of savoury and 'baked' goods, as they are known in the grocery trade, much of the naturally carbohydrate-rich ingredients like wheat flour is replaced with flour that is higher in protein and therefore lower in carbohydrate. More often than not, this is flour made from soy beans or just the protein part of ordinary wheat flour, known as gluten. They also contain fibre and other ingredients to replace the lost bulk of standard wheat flour. Ground nuts, for instance, are a favourite.

The thing to understand is that weight for weight, protein has the same calories as carbohydrate. This means that replacing wheat flour with soy flour may increase protein and decrease carbohydrate, but it does not change the calorie content of the finished food.

And here is the real irony; fat has twice the calories weight for weight compared to carbohydrate and protein. This means that when ground-up nuts are added which are high in fat, the calorie content of the finished product can be higher in calories than the original.

What appears on the label?

What often appears in bold on the labels of such foods is the boast that the food is 'Low in Carbohydrate'. This may be true. These foods are often lower in total carbohydrate. What is less obvious, however, is the small print on the nutrition panel which carries the actual calories per serving.

A slice of low carbohydrate rye bread may, for instance, only have 3g of carbohydrate compared to, say, 7g in a standard slice, but they both supply around 70 calories. Since rye bread is naturally a fairly low-GI food and will not raise blood sugar much anyway, I cannot see the point in paying the extra money for a low-carbohydrate version of this food.

I can, however, see the reasoning behind opting for a low-carbohydrate bagel. Bagels are naturally a high-GI food. This means that they raise your blood sugar levels rapidly and steeply and encourage a rush of the fat-storing, hunger-stimulating hormone insulin. A bagel that has had its rapidly digested carbohydrate reduced means that it becomes transformed into a low-GI bagel, which will keep you feeling fuller for longer. Since both the standard and low-carbohydrate bagel supply around 200 calories, in this instance it makes a reasonable choice.

The same is true of low-carbohydrate mashed potato. Standard mash is a high-GI food. Low-carbohydrate instant mash is transformed into a low GI food. The only problem is that it tastes quite, quite awful!

Low-carbohydrate sweet goods

By sweet goods I mean foods such as cakes and biscuits and chocolate products. With these foods, traditionally the main carbohydrate used in their manufacture is sugar.

When making low-carbohydrate versions of these products the sugar is removed. Obviously, it must be replaced with another ingredient that will make up for its sheer physical bulk and its sweet taste. Usually, the replacement ingredients are substances known as 'sugar alcohols' (also called 'polyols'). Sugar alcohols are a type of carbohydrate. They include maltitol, lactitol and sorbitol. Like sugar, they are sweet to taste and bulky. However, unlike sugar, they do not cause a big rise in sugar levels in the blood after eating and therefore do not raise levels of the fat-storing, hunger-stimulating hormone insulin as much. They supply slightly fewer calories, but using sugar alcohols will not make a food automatically 'low calorie'.

Manufacturers argue therefore that these carbohydrates should not 'count' as carbohydrate at all. They therefore subtract these carbohydrates from the total carbohydrates, giving a figure they describe as being 'Net Effective Carbs' or just 'Net Carbs'. Often the label says 'Low Net Carbs'.

In the small print on the nutrition information panel, the manufacturers are obliged to put in the real, total amount of carbohydrate, but it is the 'Net Carb' value which they pull out and highlight on the label and this is what first grabs our attention.

Legislative bodies in the USA are attempting to have use of this type of labelling banned, but currently it is still allowed both there and in the UK.

Low Carb Rolos and Kit Kat

If you take a look at the labelling on Low Carb Rolos and Kit Kats, you will see 'Net Carb' labelling in practice (see Table 12).

Table 12

Low Carb Rolos		Standard Rolos	
Net Carbs = 3.5g		No carbohydrate claim	
Per tube 57g		*Per tube 57g*	
Energy	200 cal	Energy	268 cal
Carbohydrate	5.9g	Carbohydrate	39g
of which sugars	3.4g	of which sugars	33.9g
of which polyols	2.4g	Fat	11.7g
Net carbs	3.5g	of which saturates	6.1g
Fat	15.2g		
of which saturates	8.9g		
Low Carb Kit Kat		Standard Kit Kat	
Net Carbs = 1.9g		No carbohydrate claim	
Per 2-bar Kit Kat		*Per 2 Kit Kat Bar*	
Energy	92 cal	Energy	106 cal
Carbohydrate	5.9g	Carbohydrate	13g
of which sugars	1.8g	of which sugars	10.4g
of which polyols	1.9g	Fat	5.5g
Net carbs	1.9g	of which saturates	3.7
Fat	6.6g		
of which saturates	4.4g		

Forget 'net' carbohydrate, the total carbohydrate is lower in the 'Low Carb' version of these well-known pieces of confectionery. But the question must be, are they really 'better' for you?

To answer this you need to study the label a little more closely.

Calories:	With the 'Low Carb' Rolos you save 68 calories, which is 'good'.
Fat:	Both the fat and saturated fats however rise slightly.

You may therefore be getting fewer calories and less carbohydrate by swapping to the Low Carb Rolos, but you are getting a higher amount of fat. How come? Because as well as using sugar alcohols to replace sugar, fat is the other ingredient often used to replace lost sugar.

The same is true for the Low Carb Kit Kat.

Calories:	You save 14 calories and almost 7g of carbohydrate by switching to the Low Carb version.
Fat:	However, again, you gain both total and saturated fats.

Apart from this nit-picking over net carbs, calories and fat, there is the simple question that rather than encouraging us to eat sweets, low carb or otherwise, would it not be more nutritious all round when choosing a regular daily snack simply to have a piece of fruit, which is packed with nutrients and supernutrients?

And if you want a piece of chocolate, rather than going for an expensive low-carb version, why not just have a piece of delicious 70% cocoa chocolate? It costs less and if you have it occasionally, it is not going to ruin your health or your figure – and because it is rich in flavonoid supernutrients, it is probably better for your heart.

Low-carb sweets

Low-carbohydrate boiled sweets and gums are more and more common. With these products most of the sugar is replaced with sugar alcohols (polyols) and no fat is added. The result is a sweet that will not raise your blood sugar as much as standard versions and so should, in theory, not set you off on a sugar roller-coaster of wanting more and more. Polyols are also less likely to cause tooth decay and so are good from this point of view.

The main problem with these low-carb sweets is that sugar alcohols are not well absorbed by the small intestine and make it down into the large intestine, where they are fermented by bacteria. During this process cramps and discomfort can occur with bloating and more often than not 'intestinal hurry' (a nice way of saying, quite simply, loose stools). All in all, it is advisable to eat these low-carb sweets in small quantities and not to give them to young children.

Sugar alcohols have half the calories of sugar, so they tend to have fewer total calories.

What is the difference?

To give you an idea of the difference in total calorie, carbohydrate and fat content of more low-carbohydrate and standard foods, have a look Table 13.

Table 13

Product	Calories	Carb g	Fat g
Atkins Low-Carb Cinnamon Raisin Bagel	200	9.0	4.0
Standard Bagel 100g	254	30.0	1.7
Atkins Peanut Chocolate Chunk Cookies	130	10.0	10
Standard Chocolate Chunk Cookies	56	6.3	2.6
Carb Options Blue Cheese Dressing 2 tbs	150	0	16.0
Standard Blue Cheese Dressing 2 tbs	100	1	9.4
Carb Options Alfredo Pasta Sauce 60g	110	2	10
Standard Carbonara Pasta Sauce 60g	98	3	8
X Carb Pork Sausages per 100g	253	0.1	23
Standard Pork Sausages per 100g	239	3.5	17
X Carb Chicken & Mushroom Soup 100g	68	2.6	4.9
Standard Chicken & Mushroom Soup 100g	53	5.7	3.0
Keto Frosted Flakes (breakfast cereal) 132g	110	9	1.0
Standard Frosted Flakes 132g	120	28	0.0

FREQUENTLY ASKED QUESTIONS

Q. *If the calories of low-carb and standard breakfast cereals are almost the same, then what is the point of buying a low-carb version?*

A. The carbohydrates in processed cereals that have a lot of sugar added are very quickly digested and leave you feeling hungry again quite soon after eating. Because the low-carb version has no added sugar, more protein and less rapidly digested carbohydrate, it will make you feel fuller for longer.

Q. *Which low-carb products replace some of their carbohydrates with fat?*

A. Foods like confectionery, cakes and biscuits tend to do this, which means that the low-carb version can end up with more calories than the standard version.

Q. *What does 'net carb' mean?*

A. 'Net carb' is a term that the makers of low-carbohydrate products have quite literally made up. They say that if a food contains sugar alcohols, since they do not raise blood sugar very much, we should not count that as carbohydrate at all. The true carbohydrate value is given on the nutrition label along with the calories per 100g serving. Always go by these figures to see what you are really eating.

And Finally ...

Low-carbohydrate labelling has no legal definition.

Net and Effective Net Value carbohydrate levels have no legal definition.

Check the total calories, fat and carbohydrate in the standard nutrition information panel. This is the only way in which you can make a fair comparison between standard and low-carbohydrate foods.

'Low carb' does not necessarily mean low in calories too.

When carbohydrate is removed from any food, it must be replaced with other ingredients. These include fat, protein and sugar alcohols.

Low-carbohydrate foods are nearly always more expensive than standard products.

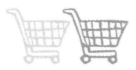

7

Pure, Natural, Traditional...
What Do These Mean?

If you have ever looked at a label and seen the words 'pure', 'natural' and 'traditional' and thought, *umm ... what exactly does that mean?*, this chapter is for you. Here are the explanations for the most commonly used expressions to help you get to the bottom of what they are all about and whether they should sway the decisions you make over the foods and drinks you buy.

Pure

You often see this one cropping up on fruit juices. 'Pure Orange Juice', for example. It should only be used on single foods to describe a single ingredient to which nothing else has been added. Pure apple juice should be just that. It should be made from pure apples.

However, that said there are odd exceptions like jam, which can be described as containing 'pure fruit', which in this context means that it has not been preserved.

Traditional

No doubt you have seen plenty of foods described as being 'traditional' on their label. Basically, the word should only be used when the food has been prepared in a way, or by a method, that is accepted as having existed for a long period of time. It could be a traditional way of making a pizza or a special, traditional way of making sausages.

Authentic

If you come across the word 'authentic' on, for instance, a 'Cantonese style' ready-made meal, it should mean that the recipe really is one that is made in this area of China. Or should you see 'Authentic Scottish Shortbread', you should be able to assume that the shortbread recipe has come from Scotland.

Home-made

There is nothing like this expression to make you think of a happy, warm, family kitchen. It should only appear on a label if the product, like a fruit cake, has genuinely been made in a domestic kitchen and is not mass-produced in a factory.

Farmhouse

Pictures of farmhouses and farmyards on a packet of, for

example, cheddar cheese are only acceptable if the cheese has actually been produced in a place that the majority of us would think of as living up to this description.

That said, it is fine for a particular type of loaf to be called a 'farmhouse' loaf (a long loaf with a split along its length), even if it has been mass-produced in a factory, because it has been called this for decades. Descriptions like 'Country Style' are frowned on and so if you do see them being used try to think objectively about the product before being seduced by the cosy image they conjure up.

Fresh

This is an interesting one! What does 'Fresh' actually mean when it appears on labels? With the exception of 'Fresh' chicken or turkey and 'Extra Fresh' eggs, there are no specific laws that dictate when it can or cannot be used.

However, the Food Standards Agency have drawn up some voluntary guidelines that they would like food manufacturers to follow, when using this word to describe their foods and drinks.

When can the word 'fresh' be used?

- Firstly, it should only be used when it has a clear meaning and can help us to distinguish between similar products. For example, a 'fresh' fruit salad should obviously be made from 100 per cent fresh fruit, and not contain slices of canned peach alongside slices of genuinely fresh apple.
- It can also be used to describe pasteurised dairy foods like

milk and cream, which have a limited shelf life. This is why you will see cartons of 'Fresh Milk' and 'Fresh Cream' in the chill cabinet.

Emotive labels

Sometimes, manufacturers like to make things a little more flowery and add extra words to further embellish the idea of a food being 'fresh' by using words like:

- 'ocean' (e.g. a piece of fish becomes 'ocean fresh');
- 'kitchen' (e.g. a 'kitchen fresh' loaf of bread)
- 'garden' (e.g. 'garden fresh' peas).

The Food Standards Agency discourages the use of these emotive words.

'Freshly cooked', 'freshly prepared', 'freshly baked'

These descriptions really do seem to add the 'ahh' factor to a food. It is hard not to feel warm and comfortable about such descriptions and they are very likely to sway a shopping decision. If it is a toss-up between 'freshly baked scones' and some plain old 'scones', I know which ones I would be tempted by.

In reality, although these labels may fire our imagination and get the saliva flowing, they may not mean anything regarding a product's quality. So if you do see these expressions, then check the period of time and context in which the claim is being used. If, for example, the scones were freshly baked on the day or morning you buy them, then that seems fair enough. If they were 'freshly baked' the day or several days before, then this is just a tad misleading!

'Freshly picked'

When you see the word 'fresh' or 'freshly picked' on vegetables and fruit, it is generally accepted in the food industry that they have not been processed. It does not necessarily mean that they have been picked just hours ago, and are still dewy from the nearest tree or bush.

'Fresh' meat

Traditionally, 'fresh' describes raw meat, as distinguished from the preserved versions. You could, for example, have a 'fresh' pork chop, whereas streaky bacon is pork that has been cured.

'Fresh' fish

It is acceptable to use the word 'fresh' when it comes to fish, if it has been kept on ice to preserve it between the time of being caught and making it to our stores. It should not, however, be used to describe fish that has been frozen and is being sold in its thawed state. The same is true for previously frozen meat.

'Freshly squeezed' fruit juice

If you pick up a carton of 'freshly squeezed' fruit juice, it does not mean that there are teams of people behind the scenes in the supermarket hand-squeezing the oranges and siphoning them into bottles. What it actually means is that you are buying juice that has been squeezed directly from the fruit rather than being prepared from juice concentrates.

Freshly squeezed juices should have a short shelf life and a date that shows they need to be drunk within two weeks of buying them.

'Freshly squeezed pasteurised' fruit juice

If a freshly squeezed fruit juice has been pasteurised to prolong the time that it lasts before going off, then the maker should tell you on his label by using the words 'freshly squeezed pasteurised fruit juice'. This is important because this kind of heat treatment will reduce the amount of vitamin C the juice contains.

If a juice has been made from juice concentrates, then the word *fresh* should not be used.

'Fresh' pasta

You would not find many makers of pasta trying to get away with using the word 'fresh' on dried forms of pasta, although you never know! Usually 'fresh' pasta is the type that needs just a couple of minutes cooking and will only last a few days in the fridge. You will find it in the chill cabinet in supermarkets and delicatessens.

'Freshly baked' bread

Unless bread has genuinely been made from scratch in the store, the use of the description 'freshly baked bread' is really not considered to be acceptable. Very often these days bread comes to the store part-baked and is then just finished off in ovens. Loaves prepared in this way should not really be described as 'freshly baked', 'baked in store' or even 'oven fresh'.

This may not matter one way or the other to you so long as your loaf is hot and tasty. But if you are a purist, then you may like to ask the store manager exactly how his bread was prepared before deciding where to buy your loaf.

Frozen 'fresh' foods

You may see the description 'frozen from fresh' on certain vegetables like broccoli or peas, or on frozen fish. This wording can be used on the label as long as the food really was frozen quickly after being harvested or caught.

Made with 'fresh' ingredients

Foods and drinks that tell you they are made with fresh ingredients should be just that! This means that they should not contain ingredients that have been dried, smoked, canned or powdered. A 'fresh strawberry milkshake' should not, for instance, have dried skimmed milk powder added or some strawberries that had been previously frozen. It should be made from fresh strawberries and fresh milk.

Equally, when a food says on its label that it has a 'fresh taste of X, Y or Z', for example of 'apples', you should expect the apple flavour to have come from real fresh apples and not artificial apple flavouring.

'Fresh' soups and sauces

Because these days there are lots of fresh soups in cartons and fresh sauces and dressings available, it is accepted that the word 'fresh' can be used to describe those that have a relatively short shelf life in chill cabinets, compared to those more heavily processed versions in cans and bottles.

Natural

If the word 'natural' catches your eye on the label, then you should be able to assume that the ingredients in the food or drink are just that – natural. In other words, that they have been produced by nature, are not man-made and do not contain additives.

It is fine for a natural food to have been baked or roasted, blanched or dehydrated, but not to have been processed any further than these straightforward techniques.

'Natural' mineral water

Bottled waters are a special category and no water can use the description 'natural mineral water' unless it complies with strict and specific regulations. If it does not meet the criteria, then it can be known as 'spring' or 'bottled drinking' water instead.

'Free from ... '

This seems like a pretty straightforward claim. 'Free from' means just that ... doesn't it? Well, actually not always.

For example, it is possible for a label to claim that a food or drink is 'free from artificial preservatives' but for it still to contain salt, which has been added for its preservative effect. And when it comes to alcohol, an 'alcohol-free' beer can still contain a little alcohol. Even though this must be less than 0.05 per cent, for someone who is alcoholic this could be a problem. The best advice when it comes to a 'free from' claim is to always look at the list of ingredients to get a balanced view of what is really in the food or drink.

'Gluten free'

Gluten is a type of protein found in wheat, oats and barley; it causes the lining of the digestive system to become badly inflamed when eaten by people with coeliac disease. This in turn leads to poor absorption of nutrients and often to malnutrition.

It is crucial that people with coeliac disease remove all traces of gluten from their diet. There are a growing number of ranges of gluten-free foods available from supermarkets these days, including biscuits and cakes, breakfast cereals and crispbreads which are made from other cereals such as maize flour and rice, and can now be enjoyed by those avoiding gluten.

Coeliac UK (*see page 251 for details*) have a full list of foods that are available for those following a gluten-free diet. It is advised that all infants under the age of 6 months be fed foods that are gluten-free. This is especially important if coeliac disease runs in the family. (*For more on this, check out Chapter 9 on Children's Food.*)

'Lactose free' and 'reduced lactose'

Some people are unable to, or find it difficult, to digest the sugar in milk called 'lactose'. The milk sugar then moves undigested into the colon where it makes the perfect food source for bacteria, which, having gorged themselves on the lactose, create gas that manifests itself as bloating and crampy pains. In some people, all lactose must be removed from their diet; for others, a certain amount can be coped with before symptoms kick in.

Milk is the main food that needs to be avoided by those with a lactose intolerance. Fortunately, there are alternatives such as soya, oat and rice-based milk and soya yoghurts, which are naturally free from lactose and usually flag this fact up on their labels. 'Reduced lactose' may also appear on some labels. There are no laws governing such claims, but the Food Standards Agency recommends that they contain at least 25 per cent less lactose than the standard product. Some actually go a lot further and contain 95 per cent less.

If you have a total intolerance to lactose, then obviously stick with lactose-free foods. If the intolerance is partial, then it is a case of trial and error as to which and how much of the reduced-lactose products can be coped with. If you have any queries about foods carrying the 'reduced lactose' claim, then contact the manufacturer and ask for specific details of the lactose content.

'Live' and 'bio'

'Live' and 'bio' are descriptions that you have no doubt seen on the labels of foods like yoghurts and yoghurt drinks. The word *bio* means 'live' in Greek and the two are interchangeable.

When it comes to their use on food, these labels actually mean very little. While they may give the yoghurt a healthy feel, there are no legal definitions controlling the use of these words. This is because all yoghurts are made by adding two types of 'live' bacteria, *Streptococcus thermophilus* and *Lactobacillus bulgaricus*, to milk to make it thicken and set. Since the yoghurts are usually then pasteurised, most of these bacteria are destroyed. In spite of this, these yoghurts can still be called 'live' or 'bio' – hence the fact that it means very little in practice!

'Bio' is often used on another type of yoghurt product that has extra bacteria added after pasteurisation. Called 'probiotic' and commonly referred to in adverts as 'good' bacteria, these cultures include bacteria with names like *Bifidobacterium bifidum* and *Lactobacillus acidophilus* which are not digested in the upper part of the digestive system.

Instead they move right through into the colon where they can grow and multiply. They are thought to help reduce problems like the bloating associated with irritable bowel syndrome and may also help to boost the immune system.

'May contain nut traces'

For anyone with an allergy to nuts it is absolutely crucial that foods containing nuts, nut oils and any traces of nuts are totally avoided. Allowing even the smallest quantity of food containing or contaminated with nuts can be life-threatening for those with a serious nut allergy.

For this reason, some manufacturers now label their foods and drinks with the words 'May Contain Nut Traces'. This is so that shoppers are aware that even though their food may seem to have nothing to do with nuts, such as jellies and ice-lollies, for example, they may actually still contain the tiniest amounts and should therefore be avoided. Often these labels are put on foods that are made on the same production line or even simply in the same factory as foods that do contain nuts. Or a food producer may add 'may contain nuts' to foods in which he cannot guarantee that the ingredients used are totally nut-free.

Anyone with, or shopping for others with a nut allergy, must take the potential presence of nuts and their derivatives extremely seriously and the advice is if in doubt, do not take the risk.

FREQUENTLY ASKED QUESTIONS

Q. *Recently, I bought some food that just had the words 'Naturally Better' flagged up on the label. What does this mean? What is the food 'naturally better' than?*

A. If you see descriptions like 'Naturally Better', 'Nature's Way' or similar, then take a step back. They really do not mean anything.

Q. *What about the supermarket 'Value' and 'Economy' ranges. Do they contain roughly the same product as the more expensive version and are they really good value?*

A. These labels do not have any official meaning but usually refer to the price of a product rather than any other inherent value. Therefore the only way to get to the bottom of what they mean is to take a bit of time in studying the ingredients and comparing one product with another.

And finally ...

Just being aware what expressions like 'Home-made', 'Farmhouse', 'Fresh' and 'Authentic' really mean can help you make more informed shopping choices.

Ultimately, if it is quality you are searching for, look beyond these descriptions and check out the product's ingredients – where it comes from and the proportions of the ingredients used.

Try to take a step back from emotive expressions and pictures used on labels. They are not always what they seem.

If you need to avoid certain ingredients in products for medical reasons, always err on the side of caution and never take a risk.

8

Symbols and Logos

These days, quite a lot of foods and drinks carry small symbols, logos and endorsements. You may have noticed a Lion Mark on your eggs, for instance, or a little red tractor on a packet of meat you are buying. These are known as 'assurance scheme' symbols. In other words, the producer is assuring you as a customer that the food has been produced to a certain standard.

In addition to these assurance scheme symbols you may also have seen logos from organizations like the National Osteoporosis Society. When a product carries such a logo, it indicates that the organization or charity is endorsing the food or drink it appears on.

You will no doubt also have come across symbols showing that a product has been given approval by, say, the Vegetarian

Society or the Vegan Society, or the Soil Association. The question is, how do producers and manufacturers go about getting permission to use one of these various symbols, and what do they mean to us?

Assurance schemes

Some of these so-called assurance schemes, such as the Red Tractor scheme, mean that the food or drink has met basic levels in the way the food has been grown and produced. Others, like the Freedom Foods scheme, mean that slightly higher standards have been met.

Basic-level assurance schemes and their logos

The red tractor

If a food you buy has a picture of a small red tractor on its label, it means that it has been produced in a way that meets British Farm Standards. This is a voluntary quality assurance scheme, and it means that the food has met the requirements of a number of bodies that set up standards regarding the way food is produced on our farms. They also regularly check that these standards are still being met.

There are ten schemes that qualify for use of the little red tractor. These include those that look into and approve the standards used to breed and rear chickens, such as the 'Assured Chicken Production' (ACP) scheme. Another scheme sets minimum standards for ways in which dairy cows are kept and fed. This is known as the 'National Dairy Farm Assurance Scheme' (NDFAS). Then there is the 'Genesis Quality Assurance' scheme, which sets standards for the rearing of beef and lamb, as well as crops.

Meeting these various standards set by the overall British Farm Standards body means that farmers have complied with basic levels of food safety, and environmental and animal welfare. Although at the moment they only have to meet basic levels of quality in these areas, a gradual increase in standards is being planned over the coming years.

Lion quality mark

If you have ever wondered what a red lion is doing printed onto your eggs, then here is the explanation. The Lion Mark scheme is run by the British Egg Industry Council. It was introduced in 1993 and updated with new rules in 1998. It guarantees to us that the egg producers who are given permission to use the symbol must have had all of their egg-laying hens vaccinated against the bacteria salmonella. Around three-quarters of all eggs produced in the UK meet these standards and carry the Lion Mark logo.

Lion Mark eggs can be traced right back to the farm on which they were laid. Along with the picture of the lion, you will find a 'best before' date so that you know when to eat them by. As well as the hens having been vaccinated against salmonella, their producers have to stick to strict levels of hygiene and animal welfare that are above the legal minimum requirements.

Danish bacon

Danish bacon that carries the words 'Danish Quality Guarantee' is one of the few quality assurance schemes from another country that are recognized in the UK. Around 1800 bacon producers in Denmark comply with the UK British Farm Standards rules for animal welfare standards; which, incidentally, are above the standards in other European countries.

When you buy bacon with the 'Danish Quality Guarantee', you know that the pigs have been bred in good welfare conditions and that the bacon meets high food safety regulations.

Symbols and logos indicating higher than minimum standards

There are some other schemes that, in terms of the welfare of animals and the horticultural production of the food, aim to meet higher levels of care than those laid down by British Farm Standards. These include the following.

Freedom Foods

The Royal Society for the Prevention of Cruelty to Animals (RSPCA) set up a scheme called Freedom Foods in 1994. The aim of the scheme was to improve the lives of as many farm animals as possible by trying to offer them freedom from fear and distress, hunger and thirst, discomfort, pain, injury and disease, and freedom to express normal behaviour. The scheme includes sheep and dairy sheep, dairy cattle, beef and pigs, hens that lay eggs, chickens, ducks and turkeys. Around 200 products bear the Freedom Foods label at the present time.

The standards are not as rigorous as organic standards. They are, however, used by big producers who are trying to raise their standards above the minimum ones laid down by law. Freedom Food standards apply to animals bred and reared both in and out of doors. Farmers, companies who transport animals, and abattoirs can only join the scheme once an assessor approved by the Freedom Foods scheme has carried out a detailed report. If they get onto the scheme, they are then regularly assessed to see that standards are maintained.

From a customer's point of view, if your food carries a Freedom Foods logo, you should be assured that the animal has had a better life than many regular farm animals. The products can also be traced back to where they were produced and you can find out who transported the animals and where they were slaughtered.

LEAF

The LEAF mark is a relatively new one that I first saw on a packet of raspberries. A leaflet positioned next to the raspberries told me that LEAF (Linking Environment And Farming) is an independent charity whose aim is to encourage farmers to produce food in a way that is friendly to the environment. People who sit on the board of LEAF represent farming groups, shoppers, supermarket bosses and conservation and environmental groups, as well as people from the food industry, education and government.

The LEAF charity helps farmers to choose the right seeds, rotate their crops and look after animals to a high standard. They encourage farmers to maintain the local landscape and countryside communities, to protect wildlife and to create a good team spirit along with everyone else involved in the scheme.

Organic logos

The Soil Association and other organic logos are types of assurance schemes. If a product carries such symbols, it means that the food or drink has been produced to certain organic standards. (*To find out more about Organic Food, turn to Chapter 10.*)

Charity health symbols

In addition to schemes that assure us of the way in which farming practices are carried out, other logos can tell us more about the finished product and how it may be particularly suitable for certain people. These include logos devised by charity organizations that license their use to manufacturers. There has been some controversy over whether these schemes mislead us as consumers, and the European Union is currently discussing whether they should still be allowed, and if so how strict the criteria must be when a manufacturer seeks permission to use one on its products.

Until this happens, it seems that the organizations and charities themselves are tightening their rules to ensure they are being responsible towards us, the consumers.

'Bone friendly' logo

The National Osteoporosis Society has created a 'Bone Friendly' logo. You will find it, for example, on orange juice and certain mineral waters that have been fortified with calcium. Osteoporosis quite literally means 'thinning of the bones'. Bones need minerals like calcium to help them reach what is known as 'maximum bone density' – in other words, to make bones as strong as possible. We need plenty of bone-strengthening minerals throughout life to keep our bones strong, and to try to slow down the natural thinning process they undergo as we get older.

To help guide us to foods and drinks which supply good amounts of the bone-building mineral calcium, the nutrition forum group of the National Osteoporosis Society grant permission for manufacturers to put their logo onto certain products which are good for calcium. The National Osteoporosis Society say that they have a strict vetting procedure and use of the logo is only granted once the nutrition forum group have agreed that the product is not only good for calcium, but is an all-round healthy food or drink. A breakfast cereal that contains added calcium but which is also pretty sugary would not, for example, be given permission to use the 'Bone Friendly' logo.

Personally, I think that the 'Bone Friendly' logo can be very useful for some shoppers, for example mums who suddenly find themselves shopping for daughters who have 'gone vegan', and are anxious to find other good sources of calcium beyond the milk and dairy foods that are traditionally great providers of this mineral.

Manufacturers have to license the use of the 'Bone Friendly' logo on their labels from the National Osteoporosis Society, which then treats the money as a donation. They specifically spend the money on educational material to help raise awareness of, and provide information and help for, people wanting to prevent and treat the disease.

The 'hummingbird' logo

Diabetes UK is the charity for people with diabetes and their overall mission is to improve the lives of these people. They provide help and support and lots of useful advice and information. This charity has a distinctive hummingbird symbol, which currently appears on leaflets and in some cookery books to show that the authors have worked in conjunction with Diabetes UK.

In the future, you may see the logo on the labels of certain foods and drinks. While the charity does not condone special 'diabetic foods', like diabetic cakes and biscuits for example, it is possible that it could appear on foods like 100 per cent whole-grain breakfast cereals. Containing no added salt or sugar, these foods are thought to be healthy additions to the diet of people with diabetes.

To get permission to use the hummingbird logo, manufacturers have to work with the charity's policy care team and pass lots of stringent tests. This means that it is not a logo that can just appear willy-nilly. If it is there on the label, it really means that the food is good for you – and that means for everyone, not just for those with diabetes.

'Tooth white' logo

This is an internationally recognized logo that is accompanied by the words 'British Dental Health Foundation Approved'. The British Dental Health Foundation is the leading UK-based independent oral health charity, which aims to help people improve their oral health. The Foundation is a charity based in the UK and a board of trustees oversees the granting of use of the smiley logo. Currently, you will find the logo on oral health products, as well as some sugar-free sweets like sugar-free mints and lollipops.

'Tooth friendly' logo

The 'Happy Tooth' logo was created on the initiative of the Institutes of Dentistry of the Swiss Universities. It helps to guide customers to foods that, quite simply, are 'friendly' to our teeth because they do not encourage tooth decay. Tooth-friendly Sweets International are keen to promote the idea that rather than ban all sweets there are some that can be eaten that do not cause cavities.

Every product that carries the logo is tested to ensure that it is 'non-cariogenic', which means that it does not cause caries, the scientific name for decay, and that it is also not erosive to the tooth. The 'sweets' that get passed often contain the natural sweetener called xylitol, that is derived from the birch tree. Xylitol helps to reduce decay-causing bacteria in the mouth and to lower acid levels. Both of these properties make it especially good at preventing decay.

Family Heart Association

The Family Heart Association has recently become Heart UK. You may find, therefore, that products that used to carry the Family Heart Association endorsement suddenly appear with a new symbol on their label. As with other charities who award the use of their logos, the vetting process is quite strict, with a nutritional advisory board having to give their permission before use of the logo is granted.

Just because a product is, for example, low in saturated fat, it does not automatically qualify. If it is low in saturated fat but high in salt, this would not be good for the heart since lots of salt in the diet raise blood pressure, which increases the chances of a heart attack.

Other symbols and logos

The Vegetarian Society 'V' symbol

The Vegetarian Society's now-famous 'V' symbol was first introduced in 1970. At first it used to appear on the society's letterheads and on window stickers in cafés and restaurants. Since the vegetarian way of life seems to have become more popular over the last few decades, an increasing number of manufacturers have actively sought permission to use the symbol as well.

To get through the vetting procedure you have to prove that your product is free from animal flesh, which includes meat, poultry, fish and shellfish, meat or bone stock, animal fats, gelatine, aspic or any ingredients resulting from the slaughter of animals. Although dairy foods are permitted, cheese which is made using the rennet derived from the stomachs of calves to separate milk into curd and whey, is not allowed. Any cheese that gets approval must therefore use vegetarian rennet. If products contain eggs, then these must be free-range eggs.

Products must be free from genetically modified organisms (GMOs) and must not have been tested on animals. In addition, to be awarded use of the 'V' symbol the manufacturer must be able to show that it is not possible for any cross-contamination with animal products to occur during production and processing. This includes all machinery, equipment, utensils, surfaces and clothing, for example.

The Vegan Society symbol

Unlike the Vegetarian Society, the Vegan Society insists that no animal products of any type can be used in products that are granted use of their logo. This means no eggs or dairy products, as well as no meat, poultry, fish or shellfish and no ingredients that are in any way derived from animal products.

They will not allow any testing on animals or any genetically modified animal genes or animal-derived substances. Although the Vegan Society symbol means that the products are suitable for people following a strict vegan diet and lifestyle, the society is keen to point out that people eating mixed diets will enjoy them just as well.

FREQUENTLY ASKED QUESTIONS

Q. *Is a 'tooth-friendly' lollipop lower in calories than a 'normal' lollipop?*

A. Usually not because they contain sweeteners such as sorbitol and xylitol, which are friendly to teeth but, like sugar, still contain calories.

Q. *Do we, the customer, pay more for foods that have a symbol or logo?*

A. No, this shouldn't be the case. Manufacturers absorb the cost of acquiring the logo and symbols.

And finally ...

Some consumer groups do not really approve much of endorsement schemes, believing that they can be confusing and misleading. The Little Red Tractor logo, for instance, may suggest that the chicken it appears on was a happy, free-range bird that ran around the farmyard, when this may not have been the case at all.

Be aware that naturally calcium-rich foods, like yoghurts, that carry the National Osteoporosis Society logo are not somehow richer in this nutrient than other yoghurts. The only difference is that one manufacturer has applied and paid for use of the logo, while another has not.

If you understand exactly what the symbols and logos mean, they can be useful. As with most food labelling, knowledge gives you the power to make informed choices and minimizes your risks of being misled.

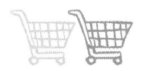

9

Children's Food

The whole issue of 'children's food' is an interesting and topical one. Recently, I've been chatting to friends about what their children eat and the overwhelming marketing of products that their children are subjected to, such as chicken nuggets and burgers, products specially designed for kiddy lunch boxes and foods like yoghurts that are plastered with cartoon characters. All agreed that these foods are very much part of our lives these days. It took a chef friend to give the subject a sense of perspective, by making the simple comment that 'children's food' is a relatively new invention.

Trotting out that old 'when I was a child' line is guaranteed to make anyone seem ancient, and yet the truth is that it was not that long ago when there really was no such a thing as food which was specially designed for and aimed at children. Maybe 'alphabetti spaghetti' and some sweets, but that really was about it.

Today, however, children's food is big business and with its growth has come lots of potential problems for our younger generation's health, in both the short and the long term. In this chapter I hope we can step back and understand why this is the case. That we can see how, through paying special attention to labels, you can help to choose foods that will be 'good' for your children, without ruining all the fun they associate with the brightly-packaged products designed to tempt them.

Baby food versus children's food – what's the difference?

Baby food

The good thing about baby food in the UK is that for babies up to one year of age there are strict laws in place that control what can and cannot be added to their infant formulas and foods. These rules help to protect babies from exposure to additives and are also there to set standards for nutritional quality.

Anyone making baby food must stick with the following rules:

- not to go over legal maximum levels of sucrose (which we know as the white or brown table sugar), fructose (fruit sugar), glucose syrups and honey;
- to have a minimum amount of protein in main meals like 'Lamb Hotpot' or 'Chicken with Rice';

- to have salt levels no higher than you would find in the food in its natural form; in other words, to contain no added salt;
- to meet the stringent maximum levels set in stone by the European Union that control pesticide levels in baby foods;
- that cereal foods intended for children under one should have minimum amounts of certain crucial nutrients, like the mineral calcium needed for the development of bones, and for vitamin B1, which helps to release energy;
- to have no colourings, flavourings, preservatives or emulsifiers added;
- to have the age of the baby for which the food is intended on the label. For example, it could state 'Not suitable for less than four months';
- if the protein gluten, found in wheat, rye, barley and oats, is present in a baby food, the label must tell us so;
- to declare the full 'Big 4 plus Little 4' set of nutritional information per 100g or 100ml, depending on whether it is a solid or liquid, and also to give this information per serving. This means that you can see how much energy the baby food is providing per serving as well as its protein, fat, saturated fat, carbohydrate, sugar, fibre and sodium content.

Children's food

The problem is that once a child reaches the age of one the laws that protect infants just vanish into thin air.

cont.

As far as foods and drinks go, once a child is one they can eat anything. Which would be fine if we all still ate the basic food that our parents and grandparents knew. Straightforward meat and two vegetables, for example, or grilled and baked fish, with home-made puddings and fruit.

Not many people eat like that anymore. Instead we often rely on processed foods which are pretty much packed with the additives that the laws forbid in foods intended for children under one.

Becoming a label detective

This is why it is even more important when shopping for children that you become a real label detective. The reason that the levels of salt and additives are restricted in foods intended for infants is because their liver and kidneys, which have to deal with detoxifying these substances, are immature and simply cannot cope. It seems a little hard to understand how, having reached the age of one, suddenly these organs are supposed to be able to manage much higher intakes. Or why, from this stage in life on, little children are fair game to be exposed to foods and drinks rich in sugar and fat.

But this is the current state of play. Which means the only way to ensure that your children are eating healthy and nutritious food appropriate for their age is to be aware of the traps into which it is easy to fall when shopping for their food.

Dodging the problem areas

- Be aware that the laws on nutrition labelling revert to those in place for all other food once your baby is over one year of age. This means that nutrition information need not appear at all. If it does it may just be the basic 'Big 4' format, giving energy, protein, carbohydrate and fat, which is often just given per 100g or 100ml, making it hard to relate it to what your child will actually eat per serving.

- Understand that manufacturers can use any permitted additives they like in children's food. This means that once your child has reached just twelve months their foods and drinks can contain lots of colourings and flavourings and any other additives used to make the food look, feel and taste child-friendly.

A survey on children's foods

If you were making a meal from scratch at home you would not have little pots of colourings, flavourings, gums, added sugars like maltodextrin and modified starches to improve its look, taste and texture.

And yet these things are common in children's food. In a recent survey of children's foods carried out by an organic baby food company called Baby Organix (BO), it was found that there was an average of five additives in each food examined. Sweets, children's desserts, cereal bars, breakfast cereals, children's drinks and frozen beefburgers contained the most.

Additives to watch out for and avoid

Colourings

Many countries have banned the use of azo dyes in foods aimed at children. Azo dyes are colours that were originally made from the processing of coal tar, but are made synthetically these days. They have been linked to triggering hyperactivity and asthma in some children.

The BO survey of children's food found that of 365 foods, a third contained colourings, with over 80 azo dyes being identified. Sweets, savoury snacks and children's desserts contained the most. One packet of cheese snacks had the azo dye called Sunset Yellow (E110), along with three other dyes to give them the yellowish, golden look. One piece of confectionery contained five azo dyes, plus two other colourings derived from coal tar that have been linked with sparking asthma and hyperactivity in some children.

The colourings listed in Table 14 are banned from children's foods in countries like the USA and in Scandinavia, and it is especially worth trying to avoid buying foods that contain them. (*Have a good look at Chapter 13 on Additives to get familiar with the names and E numbers of food colourings. The E numbers of colourings run from E100 to E180.*)

Flavourings

The word 'flavouring' covers any of the more than 4,000 flavourings allowed to be used in the making of our food and drink. Of the 365 children's foods analysed in the BO survey, 263 – that is 75 per cent – contained flavourings. Sweets,

Table 14 Banned colourings from children's foods

E102 Tartrazine
E104 Quinoline Yellow
E107 Yellow 2G
E110 Sunset Yellow
E120 Cochineal
E122 Carmoisine
E123 Amaranth
E124 Ponceau 4R
E127 Erthrosine
E128 Red 2G
E129 Allura Red
E131 Patent Blue V
E132 Indigo Carmine
E133 Brilliant Blue FCF
E142 Green S
E151 Black PN
E154 Brown FK
E154 Brown HT

cereal bars, crisps, savoury snacks, breakfast cereals, desserts, milkshakes and frozen burgers were the most jam-packed with flavourings. Flavourings do not have E numbers so there is no way of knowing which specific flavouring the food or drink contains. Reducing reliance on processed foods is the best way of reducing your children's intake.

Preservatives

Added to ensure that a food remains safe while on the shelf or in the chill or freezer cabinet, preservatives are found scattered in most processed foods. Of the 365 children's foods surveyed by BO, over 25 per cent contained preservatives. Once again, sweets contained lots, along with burgers and drinks aimed specifically at children. The E numbers of preservatives run from E200 to E285.

It is especially sensible to avoid foods that contain the preservatives which are known to trigger side effects in some children with asthma. These include sulphite, benzoate, nitrite and nitrate families of preservatives. Table 15 lists those preservatives which are to be avoided in children's foods and drinks.

Bulking-out additives

Maltodextrin, starch, modified starch and modified cornflour are added to foods to bulk them out, but while they do this job and supply energy (calories), they do not provide any nutrients. Young children need to pack as many nutrients as possible into the foods they eat, so avoid foods that are bulked up by these empty calories.

The way children's food and drink is sold to children

It is human nature to be drawn to brightly coloured foods. Fruits and vegetables fulfil the role of brightening up our

Table 15 Preservatives to Avoid in Children's Foods and Drinks

E210 Benzoic acid
E211 Sodium benzoate
E211 Potassium benzoate
E213 Calcium benzoate
E214 Ethyl 4-hydroxybenzoate
E215 Ethyl 4-hydroxybenzoate sodium salt
E216 Propyl 4-hydroxybenzoate
E217 Propyl 4-hydroxybenzoate sodium salt
E218 Methyl 4- hydroxybenzoate
E219 Methyl 4-hydroxybenzoate sodium salt
E220 Sulphur dioxide
E221 Sodium dioxide
E222 Sodium hydrogen sulphite
E223 Sodium metabisulphite
E224 Potassium metabisulphite
E226 Calcium sulphite
E227 Calcium hydrogen sulphite
E230 Biphenyl
E231 2-Hydroxybiphenyl
E232 Sodium biphenyl-2-yl oxide
E233 2-(Thiazol-4-yl) benzimidazole
E239 Hexamine
E249 Potassium nitrite
E250 Sodium nitrite
E251 Sodium nitrate
E252 Potassium nitrate

mealtimes brilliantly. Wander down the fruit and vegetable aisle of any supermarket and you will see them naturally packaged in skins that cover every colour under the sun. From the brilliant reds of strawberries and tomatoes to the purples of aubergines and blueberries, the yellow of bananas, grapefruit and sweetcorn to the orange of carrots and satsumas and the greens of everything from apples to spinach, the list just goes on.

It was through having plenty of these foods on our tables that we have brought vibrancy to our meals over the centuries. But these days it is not just fruits and vegetables that add colour to our daily diet. Colouring is used to great effect, not just in foods to make them look appetizing, but also on their packaging and their labels to stimulate, excite us and attract our attention. Food aimed at children makes absolutely full use of colour on its packaging and labelling to make sure it triggers the 'I want' button, when children nag, cajole, bargain, whinge, throw tantrums and bully their parents into putting these foods and drinks into the shopping trolley.

But it is not just brightly-coloured packaging that inspires such behaviour in children. Lots of other packaging and labelling tactics are employed by food manufacturers with great success to get us to load our cupboards with tailor-made children's food.

Once again in the label game, knowledge is power. Take a look at the ways in which food is targeted at children. Food and drink manufacturers do not leave things to chance. Many employ child psychologists to find out exactly how to turn children on. They organize what is known as 'focus' groups in which they actually test their ideas out on real children and get their opinion on what would and would not make them want to eat or drink certain products. It is not surprising that they do this – they are in the business of trying to get us to buy more food and drink.

It is only by seeing the whole picture and putting 'pester power' into context that you can make the decision as to whether you want to relent and comply with your children's demands, take the tougher route and limit it, or go the whole hog and just say no. Although difficult initially, parents I know who have taken this stance say that after a week or so it is surprising how rapidly the pestering abates. Not taking the children shopping and shopping on-line certainly make the process easier to achieve.

The marketing and promotion of foods to children

Here are some of the direct ways in which products are marketed to children on packs:

- The presence of a free gift in the packet of, say, a breakfast cereal is splashed in big letters on the packet or label.
- Famous celebrities like footballers and popstars appear on packets, along with favourite cartoon characters to capture their little fans' attention on, for example, cans of cola and packets of crisps.

Away from the actual packets themselves, manufacturers of children's foods use other tactics that dovetail in with what is found on the packaging itself:

- Foods are advertised on television and through new media like the Internet, text messaging and email newsletters, to sow the seed and then remind children that they want the food or drink concerned.
- Promotional and advertising material also uses sporting and pop heroes and cartoon characters to create the 'I want' feeling in the children's minds.
- Special on-pack promotions often tie in with schools, whereby if you collect a certain number of wrappers your school can trade them in for sports equipment, books or computers. Crisps and chocolate manufacturers are keen on these schemes.

How children's food is sold to adults

But as any seasoned shopper well knows, it is not just the 'pester power' factor from the children with which you must cope. You also have to deal with the specific marketing on packets and labels that is put there to make you think that the product is good for your child.

'Healthy' labelling

It is a natural instinct to want to feed children on nutritious foods. The problem is that it is becoming increasingly hard for us to tell which foods really are nutritious and which foods are just pretending to be so. (*Have a good look at Chapter 2 on Nutrition Labels and specifically Chapters 3 and 4 on Nutrition and Health Claims to see how manufacturers can cause confusion in these areas.*)

What about 'healthy eating' supermarket ranges for children?

It is very easy to put a healthy spin on food aimed at children by highlighting certain nutritional attributes, which may seem to be good, while blatantly ignoring the food or drink's overall nutritional contribution to the diet. At the moment it is entirely legal for a food like a fromage frais, which sports pictures of a favourite girl's doll on its packaging, to claim to be 'Low in Fat' and to have 'Added Vitamins and Minerals', when in fact it is also bursting with sugar. That said, most supermarkets do now have ranges designed for children in which sugar, fat, salt and additive levels are monitored.

What is really in children's foods and drinks?
Sugar
The recent BO survey of children's food discovered that in many cases it was impossible to find information on the sugar content in sweet foods because of poor labelling. On average, the sugar content of sweet foods was found to be almost 70 per cent, with many supplying up to 83 per cent. Children's breakfast cereals contained 36 per cent and cereal bars 33 per cent.

Fat

The BO survey discovered that fat labelling was also very poor and when it was present, few foods met the desired guideline of having less than 10 per cent of their fat coming from saturated versions.

Salt

Children are eating more than twice the Government's recommended intake of 3.5g of salt (1.25g of sodium) per day if under four, and 4.3g of salt (1.725g of sodium) if over four (see Table 5 on page 43 for guidelines on recommended salt intake). The BO survey found that the salt levels of many foods aimed at children were such that if they ate just a couple of servings of these foods that would take them way over the recommended levels. Just 20g of some savoury snacks would provide a child with 50–70 per cent of the recommended maximum intake of salt for the whole day. Many breakfast cereals, meanwhile, had 30–40 per cent of the maximum daily salt intake in just a 30g bowl.

Children's food – the survey

The survey I've quoted from above was organized by Baby Organix, a company based in Dorset, UK, that makes organic food for children. It campaigns to improve the quality of children's food and works extensively with the media and industry bodies to promote healthy eating for children.

The survey studied over 350 foods created especially for children on sale in the UK, including children's breakfast cereals, soft drinks, milkshakes, desserts aimed at children, dried fruit snacks, cereal bars and cheese. It also studied foods that children consume more than adults, such as beefburgers and savoury snacks, examining ingredients, nutritional information and the use of food additives.

(*If you would like to find out more about the survey or Baby Organix, details are in the Resource Guide.*)

Always take extra care when reading food labels for children

We are all what we eat and this is especially true for children, who are growing and developing so rapidly. Foods and drinks contain nutrients that build bones and blood, keep the heart pumping and the brain developing to its maximum capacity.

Since this is the case, do you really want your child's body to be an internal mishmash of additives? To be laden with fat and sugar? For them to develop bones and teeth that are weak, for energy levels to be on the hyper side and for excess fat to be deposited on their tummies, bottoms, arms and legs? Do you want to increase the chances of them dying before you do because their arteries have been clogged with saturated and trans fats? For their heart to have been put under so much strain through excess weight that it just gives up? For their pancreas to pack in, unable to cope with the sugar burden, which then leads to diabetes, kidney disease and blindness?

If you do not, then you really do need to be prescriptive. You need to conquer 'pester power' and buy the foods that you believe and know to be good for them. Forget people telling you that there are no such things as 'bad' foods. There are. They are packed with additives, fat and sugar and devoid of nutrients, and although once in a while a small quantity will not do any harm, the point is we do not eat small quantities any more. They have become daily features in the diets of many children and they are doing them harm in both the short and long term.

Tackling the problems

The good news is that things look as though they may be getting a little better when it comes to the promotion of implicitly unhealthy food to children. There are moves afoot to regulate the advertising of these products to children on television and to ban their sale in school vending machines. But these things will take time and when it comes to children's health, every day counts. Read the labels, resist 'pester power' and detox your own trolleys of the processed junk aimed at children.

Taking things too far

While it is a good idea to get children back to eating 'real' food, it is important not to turn them into total health freaks. Children under two, for example, should be given whole milk. Semi-skimmed is fine from ages two to five, but parents should not go mad trying to stuff them with low-fat foods that are full of fibre the whole time. Getting back to basics with simple meals and having snacks of fruit and yoghurt will help to keep the balance.

FREQUENTLY ASKED QUESTIONS

Q. *If drinks aimed at children are full of sugar, then surely they are just liquid candy?*

A. In a nutshell, yes, they are just that. A typical 500ml bottle of blackcurrant drink that has the nerve to boast on its label that it is 'rich in vitamin C' contains a shocking 70g of sugar. To give this some perspective, that is 14 teaspoons of sugar, the equivalent to the sugar found in more than three and a half packets of chewy sweets or seven lollipops. It is more than a child's recommended maximum sugar intake for a whole day. Do your children a favour, wean them off these drinks and on to water instead.

Q. *Should the advertising of junk food to children be banned?*

A. There is no doubt that advertising and marketing high-sugar and high-fat sweets and snacks to children is effective. It seems that the current code of conduct governing the advertising of food and drink products has finally been acknowledged to be inadequate, and is likely to be reviewed in the near future. Let's hope so. Until then, my advice is to minimize television viewing time in order to reduce exposure to the adverts; to leave the children at home when supermarket shopping so that they are not in the direct fire of clever marketing of products in store; and to try hard to lead by example by stocking up with and eating healthy foods and drinks at home.

Q. *Is it true that fast food chains add things to their chips to make them more tasty and therefore more appealing to children?*

A. It is true that some chains add dextrose to their chips – a form of sweet-tasting sugar that is added ostensibly to make them yellow. Then salt is often added before serving, which encourages the customer to buy more to drink to quench the thirst the salt creates. It is also wise to be aware that most fast food is specifically designed to hardly need any chewing so that it is fast to eat. The faster it is to eat, the less likely your child is to feel satisfied by it and the more likely they are to want more. It's clever marketing. My advice is to absolutely minimize trips to burger bars. Make healthy versions at home instead.

And finally ...

Never be taken in by nutrition or health claims on labels, especially when the food is targeted at children.

Always look at the list of ingredients. (*Look back at Chapter 2 which explains how to read and make sense of the nutrition label.*)

Look at the nutrition information. Remember that if a food or drink does not have any, it is probably because the manufacturer would rather that you did not know about it – in which case it is probably better if children were not eating or drinking it.

Food for infants up to one year of age must stick to strict nutritional and compositional guidelines regarding additives.

However, food aimed at children over one is totally unregulated when it comes to nutritional content and the use of additives. Many are high in fat, sugar, salt and energy.

It is crucial for parents and carers of children to take control of their children's diets and try to establish healthy eating habits for life.

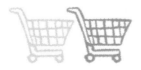

10

Organic Food

Sales of organic food have rocketed in the last decade and this trend looks set to continue. Whether you want to buy organic food for moral, environmental and/or health reasons, you need to know how to tell if a food actually is organic! And this, of course, means you rely on labelling.

The aim of the organic farmer is to produce food while maximizing the health of the environment and of the animals on the farm. In so doing, organic farmers reduce pollution and soil erosion, increase bio-diversity and sustainability and use less energy. Pesticides and artificial fertilizers are kept to an absolute minimum, as are veterinary products used in animal husbandry. As far as the consumer is concerned, the end products that we eat and drink contain, as a result, absolutely minimal residues of pesticides and herbicides.

While large studies are now under way, there is already some research that suggests that the nutritional value of organic foods may be greater than non-organic equivalents.

When is a food organic?

- To be able to call itself organic, a food or drink must have been certified organic by an independent body.
- To mention the word 'organic' in its name, 'Organic Tomato Soup' for example, at least 95 per cent of its ingredients must be organic and the label must tell you which of the ingredients are not. These non-organic ingredients can only be used because there are no organic versions of them.

Who makes the rules?

UKROFS, or the UK Register of Organic Food Standards, is the UK Government's independent body, responsible for setting, maintaining and overseeing all organic standards in the UK.

Who are the certifying bodies?

There are quite a few organizations that can certify a product is organic and award the producer the use of their certification logo. Probably the most well-known organic logo is that of the Soil Association.

The Soil Association

The Soil Association was founded way back in 1946 by a small band of farmers and scientists who were concerned about the way food was being produced and the importance of nutritious, sound soil in the production of food for both animals and humans.

As well as now being the UK's leading campaigning organic charity, the Soil Association is also the leading certification body, giving its stamp of approval to around 70 per cent of the organic food sold in the UK. Its standards are higher and more specific than those set down by UKROFS. Certification and inspection are carried out by the Soil Association's subsidiary company, the Soil Association Certification Ltd. To be awarded the Soil Association logo, farmers, growers or processors must meet the exacting standards the Association has laid down and pay a licence fee. The certification is reviewed on an annual basis so standards must be maintained.

Other organic bodies
Organic Farmers and Growers Ltd (OF&G)
If a food carries the Organic Farmers and Growers Ltd symbol, then it tells you that the food has complied with the basic organic standards set by UKROFS.

The Scottish Organic Producers Association (SOPA)
To be awarded the Scottish Organic Producers Association certification logo, Scottish organic producers must meet the UKROFS standards.

The Organic Food Federation (OFF)
This is a trade federation set up to help members, who include producers, manufacturers and importers, to market organic food. Its standards conform to those set down by UKROFS.

Biodynamic Agriculture Association (Demeter)
Biodynamic farming practices are implicitly organic but go one step further. They include planting and harvesting according to the phases of the moon and the stars. Food awarded the use of the Demeter symbol often also carries another organic certification symbol.

The Irish Organic Farmers and Growers Association (IOFGA)
The Irish Organic Farmers and Growers Association follows UKROFS standards but has additional standards of its own that producers must meet before being awarded certification and use of their symbol.

Organic Trust Ltd
The Organic Trust Ltd is a non-profit making organization. Its logo can be found on food produced and processed in Ireland.

Food Certification (Scotland) Ltd
This certification is given for organically farmed salmon that meets recognized standards. The standards are currently private because the European Union has not yet set rules.

CMI certification

CMI are a public limited company who provide a range of professional services covering food, health and safety and have recently begun to give organic certification.

International Federation of Organic Agricultural Movements (IFOAM)

This organization represents the worldwide body of organic agriculture. The Soil Association is the only UK organic certification body that is a member of IFOAM, as it is commonly known.

Which is the best certification scheme?

The Soil Association meets not just the legal minimum requirements set by UKROFS for organic farming practices, but is especially hot on standards of animal welfare, which are often higher than those required by UKROFS. In so doing the Soil Association aims to promote the highest levels of integrity in the burgeoning world of organic farming.

Are foods with the Fair Trade logo organic?

The Fair Trade logo is awarded to those who can guarantee a particular way of trading products from the developing world. They may or may not be organic. That said, Fair Trade standards do encourage environmentally friendly methods of farming. Coffee, chocolate, tea, honey, sugar and some snacks can be found in shops carrying the Fair Trade logo. (*You can find out more about Fair Trade on their website, details of which are in the Resource Guide at the end of the book.)*

Is organic food healthier than non-organic food?

Buying organic food is a way of minimizing the amount of pesticide residues that we eat in and on our food. At the moment there is only a small amount of evidence linking pesticides eaten in our diet with health problems in humans, but there is a lot linking them with health problems in animals. We do not really know what the potential toxic effects will be to us from eating pesticide residues over a lifetime, or the effect of different pesticide residues which might combine to give a cocktail effect. If you want to reduce pesticide consumption, then go for organic food. That said, the health benefits of eating standard fruit and vegetables are immense and the risk of eliminating them far outweighs the risks posed by possible exposure to pesticide residues.

Do organic farmers still use antibiotics on their pigs, hens and cows?

The routine use of antibiotics, found in standard farming practice to suppress disease and act as growth promoters, is banned in organic farming. The outbreak of disease in organic animals is reduced because they have more space and free-range lifestyles. If antibiotics are used to treat a problem, there are then strict time limits set for when the animal may be milked or slaughtered for its meat, to prevent any residues of antibiotics being found in their meat or milk.

Do organic foods contain food additives?

A wide range and large quantity of potentially harmful additives, including those that are linked with allergic reactions, are not allowed to be used in organic food production. While hundreds of food additives are allowed in normal food processing, only 30 are allowed in organic food and drink products and they can only be allowed if the producer can prove that their product really cannot be made or preserved without them. They specifically ban hydrogenated fats; phosphoric acid (found in cola); the sweetener aspartame; the flavour enhancer monosodium glutamate; and sulphur dioxide, which is used in fruit juices, soft drinks, on dried fruits, and in wine, beer and sauces. It is, however, allowed in organic wine, although the levels allowed are a third of those for non-organic wine.

Additives that are allowed to be used in organic foods
Table 16 lists the additives currently allowed to be used by manufacturers when making organic food and drink products. This list is regularly updated and reviewed.

Table 16

E160 Annatto
E170 Calcium carbonate
E220 Sulphur dioxide
E250 Sodium nitrite
E251 Sodium nitrate
E252 Potassium nitrate
E270 Lactic acid
E290 Carbon dioxide
E296 Malic acid
E300 Ascorbic acid
E306 Tocopherol
E322 Lecithins
E330 Citric acid
E333 Calcium citrates
E334 Tartaric acid
E335 Sodium tartrates
E336 Potassium tartrate
E341 (A) Monocalcium phosphate
E406 Agar
E407 Carrageenan
E410 Locust bean
E412 Guar gum
E414 Arabic gum
E415 Xanthan gum
E440 Pectin
E500 Sodium carbonates

E501 Potassium carbonates
E503 Ammonium carbonate
E509 Calcium chloride
E516 Calcium sulphate
E391 Nitrogen
E948 Oxygen

Salt or sodium chloride is used as a preservative and to enhance the flavour of foods.

Magnesium chloride, also known as nigari, is used to help coagulate soy milk when making soy-bean curd.

Organic meat and BSE

The Soil Association banned the feeding of animal protein to ruminants in 1983, five years before the Government took action in non-organic farming. Soil Association standards ban any animal not born and reared on an organic farm from being sold as organic beef. They have found no cases of BSE in any animal born and reared organically.

The nutritional value of organic fruits and vegetables

Do organic fruits and vegetables contain more nutrients than non-organic versions? This is a real hot potato. Some studies show that levels of vitamin C and the orange antioxidant pigment beta-carotene can be higher in organic potatoes and carrots. Others show minerals like calcium and magnesium are better in organic apples. More work needs to be done in this area and there are studies under way. In some ways I feel that it does not particularly matter if an organic potato has a few more milligrams of vitamin C or not. The other issues, such as pesticide residues, environmental issues and a person's moral views about whether or not to go organic, are probably much more important in the decision-making process.

Does organic food taste better?

Sometimes, but not always. Organic chicken is one food where I feel there is a big and noticeable taste difference and the same goes for organic steak and meats. With vegetables and fruit it tends to depend on the type of seed used. It does makes sense, however, that a tomato that is allowed to grow at its own natural speed, over many weeks, in nutrient-rich soil and ripen in the sun is going to be a lot tastier than one produced at breakneck speed in a greenhouse.

FREQUENTLY ASKED QUESTIONS

Q. *Why is organic food more expensive?*

A. The cost of organic food is actually coming down, although this is not always the public's perception. It is unlikely, and probably would ultimately rather defeat the object, that organic food will ever be the same price as a supermarket's standard ranges. The time, effort and investment that go into producing organic food and drink will always set it apart. This is not to say that organic food should be accessible to just the wealthy. Careful budgeting, which involves cutting back and spending less on junk food, could help open the organic market to a wider range of potential customers.

Q. *Can we trust imported organic foods?*

A. To ensure that organic products imported from other countries have been grown and produced to standards equivalent to those in the UK, the Soil Association and the International Federation of Organic Agricultural Movements, also known as IFOAM, are trying to create equivalent standards internationally. IFOAM has around 700 international member organizations in over 100 countries, with its own accreditation body that approves and accredits certification bodies in the member countries that reach its own exacting standards. Some supermarkets in the UK have signed up to a commitment to only buying IFOAM-approved organic foods from abroad. Check in your local stores where you buy your organic food to see if they follow this policy.

Q. *What is mechanically recovered meat and how do I know if my food contains it?*

A. Mechanically recovered meat is also known as MRM. It is made up from the small bits of meat that are still attached to the carcass of an animal after the prime cuts have been butchered. These bits are sucked off the bone at very high pressure. It is mostly recovered from poultry and pigs, making up to 5 per cent of the total meat that comes from a pig. It finds its way into everything from burgers to sausages and can also be used in slices of turkey, chicken or ham. If this is the case, the label has to let us know that the product has been made, or 'formed' from turkey, chicken or pork and cannot claim to be slices of these meat. You will not find this in organic meat products.

Q. *I have heard that food manufacturers can plump up chicken and meat by pumping in water. Is this really allowed and how do I know how much they have added?*

A. You will not find this in organic meat products. The label only has to declare that water has been added if it contains more that 5 per cent added water. If it is less than this, it does not need to appear on the ingredients list. Some cuts of ham have up to 25 per cent water, which is added by massaging the ham and injecting water along with additives like polyphosphates and gums. The label must tell you this.

And finally ...

🛒 Whether organic food is nutritionally better for us has not yet been fully established. But we do know organic food has fewer pesticides and residues of antibiotics. Organic food is also environmentally friendly and is produced within the highest possible standards of animal welfare.

🛒 Organic food does tend to be more expensive but costs are coming down. The more people buy organic foods, the more they will become available and the more competitively priced they will become.

🛒 Processed organic foods have been criticized for often being high in fat and sugar. As with all foods and drinks, check the ingredients and the nutrition label. Organic pies, pasties, biscuits and lemonade are just as high in calories, fat and sugar as standard versions. You still need to shop *wisely*, when you shop organically.

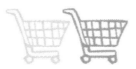

11

Genetically Modified Food

All living things – humans, animals, plants – are made up of genetic material called DNA. It is possible to selectively breed both animals and plants to enhance their good points and minimize their less desirable ones. This is a practice that has been going on in a natural way for thousands of years. The big debate raging today is over the fact that it is now possible to selectively breed certain plants by modifying their genetic material – by artificially transferring DNA from one organism to another. This is done, for example, to make a crop more resistant to insects or to a fungus that could otherwise destroy it.

Herbicides, for instance, are used to keep weeds under control in fields in which crops are grown. The problem is, these herbicides can also affect the growth of the crops they are intended to protect. The supporters of genetic modification

(GM) argue that by genetically modifying a crop by popping in a gene that makes it resistant to specific herbicides, the herbicide can then be used without damaging the growth of the crop.

Another argument in favour of genetic modification is that by altering the genetic material of a plant it can be made resistant to attack by its natural predators, like insects, and to diseases caused by infections like viruses. When it comes to animals, proponents of GM say that by altering their genes, they can be made to grow more rapidly and to a larger size.

How is GM food labelled?

If you want to avoid foods containing GM material, then European Union law has made it easier to do so since April 2004. Labelling laws now mean that the product's label has to tell you:

- all ingredients that contain or consist of GM organisms (GMOs);
- all ingredients produced from GMOs.

Exceptions to this are:

- if there is 0.9 per cent or less GM material in the food, this need not be labelled;
- there can be a presence of 0.5 per cent GM material that has not been approved for use in Europe if the European Union considers it safe;

- GM material used in some processes, like making the rinds of certain cheeses, or products from animals fed GM animal feed – which means meat and milk – do not come under this legislation and will not need to be labelled.

What are the potential problems with genetic modification?

For many people, genetic modification of our food just does not 'feel' right. We have an instinctive gut reaction that we should not be messing with nature in this way. The actual potential problems are quite complex to understand, but here are some brief pointers to give you an idea of what could go wrong when genetic modification is used in our food chain.

- In nature, many factors regulate the expression of a gene. If you take a gene out of its natural environment and plonk it in a foreign place minus these natural controlling factors, the gene may express itself in ways that could not have been anticipated.
- When physically transferring genes, things called 'gene promoters' are used, along with gene markers which help tell the scientists if the genes have been successfully transferred. The markers are often of bacterial and viral origin. We do not really know how these will impact on our health.
- As yet, there is very little safety testing on the health effects of genetically modified foods and drinks. Of the testing that has been done we do know however that, for

example, GM foods may be a problem for people allergic to soy protein or nut protein, if soy or nut protein genes have been transferred to another food and they do not know this has occurred.

How can I tell if a food or drink is made from a GM crop?

If a food or drink you are buying, for example soya-bean oil, is made from a GM crop but no genetic material is present in the oil itself, then no mention of GM will appear on the oil's label.

If, however, you are buying soya-bean sprouts that have been made from GM soya crops and GM material is present in the sprouts, which it would be, then the label would have to tell you this.

FREQUENTLY ASKED QUESTIONS

Q. *If I want to buy some cheese and it has been produced with rennin (the enzyme that makes milk separate into solid curds and watery whey) that has been genetically modified, will the label tell me so?*

A. The answer is no, the cheese producer will not need to tell you that the rennin used was GM rennin.

Q. *How will I know if the milk I am buying has come from cows fed on genetically modified crops?*

A. You won't. This applies to meat like lamb and beef that comes from animals fed on GM crops, as well as eggs laid by chickens given feed made from GM plants.

Q *Will there be some foods that will be allowed to contain GM material and not need to be labelled?*

A. Yes. Maize and soy will be allowed to contain 1 per cent GM material and not have to declare this on the label.

Q. *How will I know if the food I buy in sandwich bars, fast food places or restaurants contains GM material?*

A. At the moment, if GM material is present in your meal, then you should be made aware of this before you buy it. Detailed rules about this are currently being thrashed out at European Union level.

And finally ...

Genetic modification is a relatively new development so it is almost impossible at this stage to make any absolute pronouncements. The jury is still out on whether or not GM foods will have long-term side effects, or on how harmful or beneficial they might be.

Detailed laws governing GM foods are currently being drawn up in Europe. Until these come into play, if you want to avoid GM food, then always carefully check the label, and if in doubt opt for a food where quality is assured. *(See Chapter 8 on Symbols and Logos and Chapter 10 on Organic Food.)*

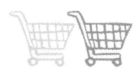

12

Functional Food

These days it is hard to find a breakfast cereal that does not have vitamins and minerals added. Look at the yoghurt section in the chill cabinet and you will find pots boasting the addition of odd-sounding bacteria. There are fruit smoothie drinks with herbal extracts and even sweets proclaiming that they contain added vitamin C.

Lobbing vitamins and minerals into foods and drinks is not a completely new thing. In fact, by law certain foods have to have nutrients added. Margarine, for example, has vitamins A and D added to bring them up to the levels found in butter. And white flour used for bread-making has the minerals and vitamins lost during milling, which include calcium, iron, vitamin B1 and niacin, added back in. This is a throwback to the Second World War when the fortification was crucial to the health of a nation living on war rations. Similarly, infant milk formulas must also be fortified with various nutrients to try to make it as similar as possible in composition to breast milk.

Adding voluntary extras

These exceptions aside, other fortification is voluntary and is usually done to give the manufacturers something to boast about on their labels and to make their product different from others on the shelves. These 'added value' products are often described as 'Functional Foods'.

There is no legal definition in the UK as to what a functional food is. They are usually described as being foods that give a health benefit beyond the basic nutrition they supply.

'Functional' margarine

Some new types of margarine have more than just vitamins A and D added. They are also topped up with substances called plant stanol and plant sterol esters.

Plant stanol and plant sterol esters are natural substances found in certain plants. They are not absorbed in the digestive system but pass out undigested in the stool. They have one important action in the digestive system, however, and this is their ability to grab hold of cholesterol. They then keep hold of it and both they and the cholesterol get passed out of the body in the stools. This means that instead of the cholesterol being

cont.

reabsorbed into the blood, it is eliminated from the body and blood levels of cholesterol fall.

This type of margarine has gone beyond the role of being a spread that supplies us with fat and vitamins A and D, and has taken on the additional role of actively reducing cholesterol. The same is true of yoghurts containing these plant stanol and plant sterol esters.

Because these kind of foods have been thoroughly researched and have definitely been shown to lower blood cholesterol in people whose levels are raised, they are allowed to make a specific health claim declaring: 'This spread contains a unique ingredient called plant stanol ester which can actually help to lower cholesterol as part of a healthy diet'. (*See Chapter 4 for more on Health Claims.*)

Functional foods abroad
America

In America there are laws that allow producers of such foods to make direct claims about their health-giving, disease-preventing properties if they can back up the claims with hard science. So far in America there are 13 specific health claims that have been approved for use on 'Functional Foods' and dietary supplements.

Japan

Japan is even further ahead. 'Functional Foods' are a well-established section of the Japanese food market. Under

Japanese law, manufacturers can make specific claims about a food on the label, if that food is able to remedy a serious health problem. The Japanese government makes it quite clear that they support these kinds of added-value, health-promoting foods, in the hope that by encouraging people to eat and drink them they can improve dietary habits and so cut the cost of health care.

The UK
In the UK, with the exception of the odd specific claim, all other 'Functional Foods' and drinks that have not been given special permission to make a claim must follow the general guidelines that cover health claims on food. (*See Chapter 4 on Health Claims.*)

Are They Good for Us?
There is general agreement that in some cases the extra nutrients, supernutrients, good (probiotic) bacteria, and in some cases standardized herbal extracts popped into certain foods and drinks may be beneficial for some people.

The key is to get the balance right. What is the point of tucking into a packet of sugar-rich sweets containing added vitamin C when you could have an orange instead, and get the vitamin C minus the added sugar?

Too much of a good thing?
One concern is that with nutrients added left, right and centre to foods and drinks, we could end up having too much of certain vitamins. Take vitamin A. Pregnant women need to be

careful not to have more than 700 µg a day. Although the level of intake at which a relationship with birth defects has been found is 3,300 µg a day, it is best to stick to no more than the recommended nutrient intake of 700 µg a day. Not to do so may damage the unborn baby.

Other nutrients, like vitamins B6 and D, nicotinic acid and zinc, can be toxic if you go above upper safe limits.

Typical Functional Ingredients
Good bacteria
What are they?
You will find bacteria with long, tongue-twisting names like *Lactobacillus casei Shirota* or *Lactobacillus plantarum 299v, Lactobacillus johnsonii* and *Lactobacillus casei Immunitas,* splashed on labels on yoghurts, yoghurt drinks and even fruit drinks.

What do they do?
These are bacteria that avoid digestion and travel down into the colon where they multiply. They help to reduce the number of bad, disease-causing bacteria and seem to help boost the immune system. Some research also shows that these good bacteria can help to improve symptoms of irritable bowel syndrome (IBS). When taking antibiotics the natural balance of bacteria in the colon can be disturbed. Having probiotics in foods and drinks may help to restore this balance, improve digestive health and boost immunity.

What claims can actually be made for them?

Labels often carry quite wishy-washy health claims such as: 'Help your body protect itself from the inside', or 'Taken daily, these friendly bacteria help maintain a favourable balance of bacteria in the digestive system. A healthy digestive system helps promote overall well-being'.

What's the verdict – are they good for you?

If you have foods and drinks supplying these good bacteria on a daily basis, they may well help to give your immune system a boost and improve problems, such as bloating, associated with IBS.

Essential fats

What are they?

These are essential fats called 'Omega-3' fatty acids that are usually found in oily fish like salmon, mackerel and sardines, anchovies, pilchards and, to a lesser extent, tuna fish. Dark green vegetables, rape and linseed oils, walnuts and flax oil contain a type of fatty acid that can be converted into these essential fats. You can now find loaves of bread, spreads and eggs containing Omega-3 fats in the supermarket.

What do they do?

There are two important Omega-3 fatty acids, EPA and DHA. Research shows them to be of crucial importance to the development of the brain in babies in the last three months of pregnancy and the first months of life. A lack of them has been associated with problems such as dyslexia and hyperactivity in children, and depression in adults. They have also been shown to help reduce the risk of blood clotting and to reduce inflammation, helping to improve symptoms of rheumatoid arthritis, psoriasis and Crohn's disease.

What claims can actually be made for them?
'Rich in Omega-3, which can help protect the heart', 'May play a part in the maintenance of a healthy heart and circulation.'

What's the verdict – are they good for you?
Our intake of Omega-3 essential fats does seem to have fallen during the last century due to a reduced consumption of oily fish. We only eat 0.1g a day and the Government recommends doubling this. Increasing our intakes can do no harm and may well be extremely beneficial for both adults and children who do not regularly eat oily fish.

Plant stanol and plant sterol esters
What are they?
Plant stanol and plant sterol esters naturally exist in plants and are now added to certain brands of margarine and yoghurt.

What do they do?
They have been shown to help lower cholesterol in the blood by latching on to cholesterol in the digestive system and carrying it out of the body in the stools.

What claims can actually be made for them?
These ingredients are allowed to make a specific claim: 'This spread contains a unique ingredient called plant stanol ester which can help to actually lower cholesterol as part of a healthy diet.'

What's the verdict – are they good for you?
If you have raised LDL (bad) cholesterol, then using products containing plant sterols and stanols may well help to lower it. If you do not have raised cholesterol, then they are not worth the extra money you have to pay for them.

Calcium

What is it?
Calcium is a mineral that is crucial for the building and maintenance of strong bones and is also needed for the contraction and relaxation of muscles. It is naturally found in dairy foods like milk, yoghurt and cheese; in oily fish eaten with its bones like canned sardines; in nuts, sesame seeds, dried fruits and in dark green leafy vegetables like cabbage. It is now also found added to orange juice and mineral water and foods like breakfast cereals and breakfast bars.

What do these calcium-enriched foods do?
They supply extra calcium.

What claims can actually be made for them?
That they 'Build and maintain strong bones'.

What's the verdict – are they good for you?
For people who do not get sufficient calcium from foods
naturally rich in calcium, they can make a really helpful addition
to the diet. The only problem is that some products, like sugar
and salt-rich breakfast cereals and sugar-loaded breakfast bars,
are not exactly all-round healthy foods. You need to choose
carefully when deciding to use calcium-enriched foods and
drinks to boost your levels of this mineral.

Added plant oestrogens

What are they?
Plant oestrogens are naturally found in foods like soya and
lentils. They are now being added to things like loaves of bread.

What do they do?
Plant oestrogens are 'supernutrients' which are very similar in
shape to human oestrogen. They therefore have an ability to
latch on to oestrogen receptors in the body – in the breast
tissue of women and in the prostate of men, for example. By so
doing they may seem to reduce the risk of human oestrogen-
triggered cancers, like breast and prostate cancer. They also
seem to have a role to play in lowering symptoms of the
menopause, like hot flushes, and improving bone health
through imitating the role of human oestrogen.

Foods enriched with plant oestrogens may play a role in helping to reduce certain cancers and improve symptoms of the menopause.

What claims can actually be made for them?
'A rich source of plant oestrogens.'

What's the verdict – do they work?
No one really knows. They will probably not do any harm, though, and may well be beneficial. Or you could instead just try drinking soy milk, eating soya-bean curd (tofu) and having lots of pulse vegetables, which are natural sources of plant oestrogens.

Energy boosters
What are they?
These are soft, sugary drinks, both sparkling and still, that supply extras such as caffeine, vitamins, herbs and taurine.

What do they do?
They provide energy (calories) in the form of sugar as does any other soft non-diet drink. Sometimes this is in the form of glucose rather than sucrose (table sugar). They give the impression that they stimulate you, give you energy and boost concentration.

What claims can actually be made for them?
They get away with saying things like: 'Designed to boost alertness' and 'Stimulates metabolism'.

What's the verdict – do they work?
Many of these drinks supply around 7–9 teaspoons of sugar so they will definitely give you energy. But then so would a piece of fruit or a glass of fruit juice. The caffeine they contain is a well-known stimulant and you could easily get it from a cup of strong coffee. There is a lack of evidence that the other things that some also contain, such as ginseng and royal jelly, are going to do any real good.

Soy protein

What is it?
Some foods are now having soy protein added to them. Breakfast cereals and some biscuits, for example.

What does it do?
There is pretty good evidence that the protein in soy helps to lower bad 'LDL' cholesterol. An intake of 25g a day is thought to have this cholesterol-lowering effect.

What claims can be made for these products?
Like plant stanol and plant sterol esters, specific health claims can be made: 'Helps maintain healthy cholesterol levels' and 'Soy protein helps maintain a healthy heart'.

What's the verdict – does it work?
It would seem from the current research that tucking into foods with added soy protein may well help to lower raised levels of bad cholesterol and may in turn, therefore, help to reduce the risk of heart disease. You could just eat lots of soy food like soya-bean curd (tofu) and soy milk and yoghurts, but the foods enriched with soy protein give you added choice.

Other functional foods

Detox smoothies
Some fruit smoothies add herbal extracts such as milk thistle and imply that they will help us to detox. There is evidence that 'standardized extracts' of this herb help the liver to repair itself. It depends on the amount consumed, how often it is consumed and whether we are able to absorb it in the form found in such drinks, as to whether the drink actually has the promised effect.

What is a 'standardized extract'?
This means that the active or main ingredient is carefully controlled so that it does not vary from batch to batch of the supplement you buy. For example, with milk thistle you would want to buy a product that has '80 per cent silymarin'. If a herbal supplement does not give the standardized extract, then it is likely that the levels vary widely between bottles and batches, and then who knows how much you are actually getting of the active ingredient?

Sugar-free sweets with vitamin C

Well, at least they are free from sucrose (table sugar), which can reduce the risk of tooth decay. An intake of 50g worth of such sugar-free sweets can supplies over 200 per cent of the daily recommended amount of vitamin C, so they certainly provide a good slug. The only problem is that the isomalt used to replace the sugar can have a laxative effect when eaten in the amounts found in 50g of sweets. You are probably better off sticking with an orange and other foods like kiwi fruit, berries, peppers and dark green vegetables for your vitamin C.

Foods with prebiotics

Prebiotics provide food for probiotic (good) bacteria in the colon. They include inulin, a type of carbohydrate found naturally in chicory and bananas and now added to some yoghurts. Foods containing both pre- and probiotics may well be useful if you have an upset tummy or are taking a course of antibiotics, as these tend to disturb bacterial balances in the colon and in doing so may lower immunity.

Milk to make you sleep

This is a slightly unusual one because rather than having anything added, some milk is now available that comes from cows who have been milked at a certain time in the morning to ensure that their milk contains higher than usual levels of the hormone melatonin. The producers of this milk claim that because mela-tonin is a natural substance that regulates our body clock, it will help to trigger the desire to sleep. The jury is out on this one.

Eggs that are naturally rich in Omega-3 oils

These, which claim to protect the heart, are a similar case to the milk that is naturally rich in melatonin. The chickens' feed is rich in Omega-3s, so therefore their eggs are.

Q. *What other sorts of functional ingredients might we expect to see in the future?*

A. It is possible that in the future we may find foods and drinks on our supermarket shelves that contain things like added collagen, designed as a nutritional approach to anti-ageing; or that mushroom extracts may be added to foods to reduce bad breath. Green tea antioxidants could be added to drinks to help control allergies, and antioxidants to reduce eye strain. The way forward for functional foods is currently wide open. The area is in desperate need of strict regulation and rules to ensure that it does not go so completely potty that we hardly have any real foods left.

Q *If I eat breakfast cereals, fruit juices and cereal bars, all with added vitamins and minerals, am I at risk of overdosing?*

A. It is possible to have too much of a good thing – even vitamins and minerals. I would be very wary of overdoing foods with added nutrients, especially when it comes to children. Personally, I think if you are going to allow any at all, it is worth sticking to one product category, such as breakfast cereals, and avoiding other products with vitamins and minerals for the rest of the day.

Q. *Are there any really useful functional foods on the market at the moment?*

A. Products with plant stanol and plant sterol esters do seem to help reduce cholesterol in people who have raised LDL or 'bad' cholesterol. Equally, mineral waters and orange juice with added calcium can be useful if dairy intakes of this important bone-strengthening mineral are low. I also feel that foods with probiotic 'good' bacteria can be useful for strengthening immunity and restoring balance to the colon, especially while taking antibiotics. And foods with Omega-3 oils are great for people who eat little oily fish. Otherwise, at the moment I think that functional foods should be treated with caution. I would recommend buying and consuming them only if you really know that they will be of benefit to your health and they have no nutritional downsides. Added nutrients being consumed within an implicitly unhealthy food, like a sugary drink or chocolate spread are not a good idea.

And finally ...

Firstly, make sure that the 'Functional Food' is a healthy food from a holistic perspective. Do not get tempted by an energy-boosting drink that contains guarana and caffeine, for example, if it is also packed with sugar. You may as well just have a cup of coffee.

Next, consider what you or your family may particularly benefit from. If you have a family member with raised cholesterol, it is worth considering buying foods with added extras that specifically lower cholesterol, like margarine with plant stanol or plant sterol esters and foods with added soy protein. If you have few dairy foods, then drinks with extra calcium may be helpful.

Be selective, because buying them for no particular reason will not necessarily benefit your health but will definitely cost you more on your food bill.

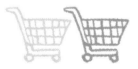

13

Additives

Mention the word 'additive' and most of us conjure up images of bright orange colourings that send children into a whirling frenzy of hyperactivity. But the term additive covers more than just colouring agents. The list of extras that can be mixed into our processed foods is pretty long. They fall into several different categories and are added by manufacturers to foods for a variety of reasons.

One category, preservatives, is obviously added to protect food from going off, which means it can stay on the supermarket shelves for longer and remain safe to eat. Other additives are put into foods and drinks to make them more tasty, to make them look nicer or, for example, to make them thicker or prevent them from separating or getting clogged up.

Types of food additives

Acidity regulators
These substances help to control the level of acidity in a food or drink. They may help to maintain, for example, the sharp acidic flavour of lemonade.

Anti-caking agents
These literally stop things like dry powdered cake mixes or baking powder from forming into clumps.

Anti-foaming agents
While drinks like beer need a foam to taste good, you can have too much of a good thing. Anti-foaming agents stop it from becoming one big froth. Jams also contain anti-foaming additives based, for example, on silica gel.

Antioxidants
Foods rich in fat, like sausages and vegetable oils, go rancid if left to their own devices. Antioxidants slow down this process. Vitamin E is an especially effective antioxidant and is found added to many foods, including margarine.

Bulking agents
Found in everything from ice cream and milk shakes to frozen mousses, cottage cheese, dips and spreads, bulking agents add bulk to foods without adding loads of calories. Cellulose, a non-digestible fibre, is a good example of a bulking agent.

Colourings

There are three types of colours used in foods. There are natural colours, like the bright orange beta carotene from carrots, or the red colour cochineal from the female Coccus cacti beetle; there are so-called 'inorganic pigments' made from metals like silver; and finally there are synthetic 'azo' dyes like the yellow colouring quinoline yellow. Azo dyes used to be made from coal tar but are now made completely from scratch by scientists in laboratories. They are called 'azo' because chemically they contain something called an 'azo' group.

Emulsifiers

Oil and water usually do not mix together. The way to get them to do so is to add an emulsifier. When making a mayonnaise, cooks get oil and the watery part of vinegar to hold together by adding an egg. It is a substance called 'lecithin' in eggs which has this power to keep the two ingredients held together in an emulsion. Lecithin is a type of emulsifying agent used in food manufacturing, along with others like the albumin in eggs and agar from seaweed. Emulsifiers are found in foods like margarine and ice cream, salad creams and mayonnaise. They are also found in some baked goods, like cakes.

Emulsifying salts

These are substances that are added to foods like evaporated milk, milk powder and processed cheese to keep them stable and 'together'.

Firming agents

In nature, foods like strawberries and other fruits contain a type of jelly-like fibre called 'pectin' which helps to keep them plump and firm. Firming agents are used in food production to help retain this kind of firmness or crispness when they are being processed. They are added, for instance, to pulses like red kidney beans when they are being canned, and to red cabbage so that it stays crunchy even when pickled.

Flavour enhancers

These additives do what they say – they perk up the flavour of other substances in foods and drinks although they do not have any characteristic flavour of their own. The best-known flavour enhancer is monosodium glutamate. It can be found in savoury snacks, pork pies, packet soups and many more foods.

Flavourings

There are over 4,000 flavouring agents used in food but when it comes to the label the manufacturer only has to write the word 'flavourings' – the specific chemical name does not have to be given. There are four main types of flavourings allowed in the UK. These are natural flavourings, a mix of natural and synthetic flavourings, smoke flavourings made from smoke extracts, and flavours which are totally created by chemists and are not found anywhere in nature.

Flour treatment agents

To keep white flour white or make a flour less 'strong', and suitable for cake- rather than bread-making, things like sulphur dioxide or vitamin C and nitrogen peroxide are added to flour.

Foaming agents

These additives do the opposite of anti-foaming agents and encourage foam in foods and drinks to form.

Gelling agents

Agar, which comes from seaweed, and carob gum from the carob bean are both natural substances that create gels. They can be found in the jelly part of trifles, in salad creams and in some ice creams.

Glazing agents

Glazing agents give food an appetizing and appealing shiny surface and a polished look. In some cases, as well as being used to make a food look nice, the glazing agent may have a protective role as well.

Humectants

These additives help to absorb moisture in a food, which in turn helps to stop the growth of moulds. For example, glucose syrup and honey, as well as sorbitol, are humectants and are used in things like ready-made cakes. Another, glycerine, can be found in royal icing.

Modified starches

Starches which have been altered by various chemical or physical treatments to give them a special use in food processing are called 'modified starches' and you will find them all over the place in foods and drinks. Sometimes the starch may be processed further to alter its clarity, or be treated with acid to reduce the stickiness of a paste used in making sweets, like gum drops and jelly beans.

Packaging gases

These are gases that are pumped into the packaging of products like ready-prepared salad leaves, to stop them going brown.

Preservatives

Foods go off because micro-organisms like bacteria and fungi take hold and start growing on and in the food. Foods also go off through the action of oxygen – a process called oxidation. A good example is a cut slice of apple going brown when exposed to oxygen in the air. In addition, enzymes naturally present in a food can make it go off. Preservatives basically are used to protect food from these processes. In the old days salting, smoking, drying and pickling were common methods of preservation. Freezing and canning and modern processes are now used to preserve food. There are 30 preservatives allowed in our foods and drinks. They include chemical substances like sulphur dioxide, which is used to coat dried fruit like apricots, to stop bacteria from growing. As well as chemicals like benzoic acid, which may be added to beer and fruit juice, fruit yoghurts and dessert sauces, natural preservatives include salt, sugar and vinegar.

Propellants

A product that comes in an aerosol, such as a can of whipped cream, needs a propellant to push it out. Propellants come in the form of gases or volatile liquids that are released when a button is pressed.

Raising agents

Baking powder or 'sodium bicarbonate' is one of the best-known raising agents and is used both in home cooking and food manufacturing to help foods to rise. When moistened or heated, it releases carbon dioxide that gives the raising effect. Scones are a typical food that can contain raising agents.

Sequestrants

Traces of metals like iron and copper occur naturally in food and can cause the food to oxidize and go off prematurely. Sequestrants are substances that latch on to these traces of metals and make them inactive.

Stabilizers

Emulsifiers and thickeners like agar and carob gums can also have a slightly different role as stabilizers, helping, for example, to stabilize and maintain the texture of meringues and marsh-mallows, and even bread.

Sweeteners
There are two types of sweetening agents that can be added to foods. Saccharine and aspartame, for example, are used in tiny, tiny amounts, have no calories and are known as intense sweeteners. Bulk sweeteners are various types of bulky sugars including sorbitol and isomalt and they are used to replace sugar in foods like sugar-free boiled sweets and chewing gum.

Thickeners
These additives are equivalent to adding flour to a sauce or gravy at home to make it thicker. They often come from plants. Guar gum is a good example of a thickening agent; it comes from the cluster bean, a member of the pea family, and is used in foods like ice cream and milkshakes, horseradish cream and salad dressings.

Where do all these additives come from?
Quite a list, isn't it?! Within each category there are lots of individual additives which are designated with an E number, giving a total of more than 500 different ones that are legally allowed to be added to our foods. In addition to this, there are approximately 4,000 flavours that can be used that do not have an E number.

Many additives are, in fact, natural. While they are there to specifically perform one role, some also give added important nutritional benefits – like vitamin E, which is used to stop a vegetable oil going rancid. Obviously, having a little more of this essential vitamin is a good thing. Another example is lycopene, the red colour in tomatoes, which is used to colour foods red;

it is also thought that high intakes may help to reduce the risk of problems like heart disease.

What is an E number?

With the exception of flavours, additives that are given the OK by the European Union are given an E number. They have got themselves a pretty bad name over the last few decades and, being aware of this, food manufacturers often now just list the full name of the additive and leave off its E number, in the hope that we will not be put off their food or drink.

Yet the point is that an E number reflects the fact that as far as the European Union are concerned the substance has been proven safe to use in food processing. The whole subject is a movable feast; if evidence mounts up against an approved additive, it can have its E number removed and will no longer be allowed to be used.

Maximum permitted levels

There are 'Maximum Permitted Levels' of the individual additives allowed in foods that are based on 'Acceptable Daily Intakes', or ADI. An ADI of an additive is the amount that can be taken on a daily basis over a lifetime without damaging health. The ADI depends on your weight and age. People, especially children, who drink a lot of fizzy drinks that are packed with colourings and sweeteners may risk going over the ADI for some of these additives.

Obviously, not all of these additives are packed into every food we eat. But it may surprise you to learn that so many are legally allowed now, it has been estimated that over the course of a year we tuck away around three kilograms of additives. Generally, we will always know exactly which additives are in our food. The exception is with flavourings, where manufacturers do not have to specify which ones have been added.

Are additives a good or bad thing?

This depends on your individual view. If you are a food manufacturer, then obviously they tend to be a good thing. Although only a very small proportion of additives used are preservatives, the other additives like flavour enhancers and emulsifiers, anti-caking agents and substances that make your product more bulky are a great advantage. They make it possible to produce an ever-expanding array of brightly-coloured, 'tasty' foods that can remain on the shelf for long periods of time. Many modern foods simply would not exist without the use of additives to create their physical structure, taste and colour.

Some shoppers would certainly consider this to be an advantage and would rather have such foods with the additives they implicitly supply. Other shoppers are aware that some additives may pose health risks and they actively avoid foods and drinks containing them. If you know that you or a member of your family are intolerant of certain foodstuffs or can suffer bad reactions to certain preservatives, they are not such a great thing. A list of the additives most often associated with adverse side effects is provided later in this chapter.

How can I minimize my intake?

If you want to minimize the amount of additives you eat because you instinctively just do not like the idea of swallowing hundreds of added chemicals, then you have to go back to basics. This means cutting out all standard processed foods, and by that I mean all ready-made meals, sweets, cakes, biscuits, squashes, fizzy drinks, jam, mustard and so on. You have to stick with fresh cuts of organic meat, chicken and fish, and fresh and frozen vegetables and fruit.

Being aware of why and how additives are used in food and drink production allows you to stand back and think objectively about whether you personally want them as part of your diet and life. Once you know the roles they play you can decide if, for example, you would prefer your dried apricot coated in sulphur dioxide to keep its raw orange colour, or an uncoated version which is dark brown, the real colour of dried apricots. It is your choice as to whether you buy plain yoghurt and add real strawberries to it, or you buy a strawberry-flavour yoghurt that contains additives to give it a pink colour and strawberry taste.

Criticism over such extensive use of additives in food tends to focus on the fact that some are thought to be linked with adverse reactions and that they are sometimes used to disguise the use of cheap ingredients; for example, burgers that contain cheap, fatty cuts of meat but are made to look and taste better with red colourings and meat flavourings. However the burgers may look and taste, to the body they are still fatty bits of meat.

Which additives may cause unwanted reactions?

Allergic reactions, asthma and hyperactivity

Azo dyes

- While all the azo dyes have an E number and are therefore considered to be safe by the European Union, there is anecdotal evidence that many of them, such as E102 Tartrazine, E104 Quinoline yellow, E110 Sunset yellow, E122 Carmoisine, E123 Amaranth, E124 Ponceau, E128 Red 2G and E155 Brown HT can trigger asthma, skin rashes and rhinitis (which results in watering eyes and a runny nose), blurred vision and purple patches on the skin. They are also linked with hyperactivity in some children.

- Scientists say that there is uncertainty about whether food additives are linked to adverse effects on behaviour and that a lot more research is needed to prove things one way or the other. If you think that you or someone you know does react badly to azo colourings in food, then the best advice is to make sure that you avoid them.

Preservatives

- E210 Benzoic acid, E211 Sodium benzoate, E212 Potassium benzoate, E213 Calcium benzoate, E214 Ethyl 4-hydroxybenzoate and E215 Sodium ethyl p-hydroxybenzoate, E217 Sodium propyl p-hydroxybenzoate may trigger asthma and urticaria.

- All sulphites, including E221 sodium sulphite, E222 Sodium hydrogen sulphite, E223 Sodium metabisulphite, E224

Potassium metabisulphite, E226 Calcium sulphite, E227 Calcium hydrogen sulphite and E228 Potassium hydrogen sulphite, can trigger attacks in people with asthma by causing the airways to become tight and constricted; they should therefore be avoided.

- Foods for babies less than six months old should not contain added nitrates as they can lower the ability of the blood to carry oxygen.

Antioxidants
- All alkyl gallates which include E numbers (E310 Propyl gallate, E311 Octyl gallate and E312 Dodecyl gallate) may cause problems for people with asthma and those sensitive to aspirin.

Kidney problems
- E173 aluminium is absorbed by the digestive system and should be eliminated from the body via the kidneys. People with damaged kidneys may find it more difficult to eliminate, therefore it would probably be advisable for them to avoid the cake decorations which contain this E number.

Skin irritants
- Some preservatives, like E200 Sorbic acid, may trigger skin irritability. E216 Propyl p-hydroxybenzoate, E217 Sodium propyl p-hydroxybenzoate, E218 Methyl p-hydroxybenzoate and E219 Sodium methyl p-hydroxybenzoate may irritate the skin and have a numbing effect on the mouth.

- E321 Butylated hydroxytoluene may trigger skin rashes in some people.

Irritation of the digestive system and gastro-intestinal problems

Certain preservatives may also trigger gastro-intestinal problems:

- E223 Sodium metabisulphite, E 220 Sulphur dioxide and other sulphites E221–E228 can cause irritation in the stomach lining because they release sulphurous acid.
- E252 Potassium nitrate may cause stomach pains and vomiting.
- The bulk sweetener E420 Sorbitol may cause problems with flatulence, diarrhoea and bloating if too many foods containing it are eaten.
- E421 Maitol may cause nausea, vomiting and diarrhoea in particularly sensitive people.
- E627 Disodium guanylate, E631 Disodium inosinate and E635 Disodium 5'-ribonucleotides may be a problem for people with gout. They are flavour enhancers found in pre-cooked dried rice snacks, crisps and gravy granules.

Headaches

- The flavour enhancer E621 Monosodium glutamate is reported by some people to cause dizziness and headaches.

Additives unsuitable for babies and children
(Also see Chapter 9 on Children's Food)

- E249 Potassium nitrite should not be given in foods or drinks to babies under six months of age.
- All alkyl gallates which include E numbers, E310 Propyl gallate, E311 Octyl gallate and E312 Dodecyl gallate, should not be used in foods intended for babies and young children.
- Similarly, E320 Butylated hydroxyanisole and E321 Butylated hydroxytoluene should not be used in foods intended for babies or young children.
- E621 Monosodium glutamate is not suitable for children and young babies.
- E627 Disodium guanylate is prohibited from use in foods intended for young children and babies.
- E631 Disodium inosinate is banned from foods made for babies and young children.
- E635 Disodium 5'-ribonucleotides is not allowed in foods for babies and young children.

And finally ...

It is hard in this day and age to totally avoid eating food and drinking drinks that contain additives. It is, however, possible to minimize intakes.

The most effective way of doing so is to eat organic food or simply to go back to eating the way our grandparents would have done – with traditional 'meat (or fish, or other protein) and two veg' type meals, along with plenty of fresh fruit and vegetables.

By cutting right back on processed foods, snacks, sweets, shop-bought cakes and biscuits, you can really reduce your additive load.

Personally, I think any change you can make to your diet that reduces the reliance on over-processed food, which by its nature requires lots of additives to give it form, taste, texture, colour and preservative qualities, is a step in the right direction.

Additives: a quick guide

Some additives appear in more than one group but Table 17 provides an at-a-glance guide to the E numbers of different groups of additives.

Table 17

Colours	E numbers 100–180
Preservatives	E numbers 200–285
Antioxidants	E numbers 300–321
Sweeteners	E numbers 420–421 and 953–959
Emulsifiers, stabilisers, thickeners and gelling agents	E numbers 400–495

Others

E numbers given a number of 500 plus include the other additives such as: acid regulators, anti-caking agents, anti-foaming agents, bulking agents, firming agents, flavour enhancers, foaming agents, humectants, modified starches, packaging gases, propellants, raising agents, carrier solvents, emulsifying salts, acids and sequestrants.

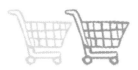

Appendix:
Permitted E Numbers

Colours

E100 Curcumin
This is a natural colouring that is extracted from the root of the turmeric plant. It gives foods an orange-to-yellow colour. Curcumin is found in curry powders, processed cheese, savoury rice and margarine.

E101 (i) Riboflavin
Made naturally from yeast as well as synthetically, riboflavin, also known as vitamin B1, has a yellow colour which it imparts to food. It is typically found in processed cheese.

E101 (ii) Riboflavin-5'-phosphate
Known as vitamin B2, this vitamin also has a yellow colour. It is made synthetically for use in foods like yellow and orange coloured jam.

E102 Tartrazine
An azo dye with a vibrant and strong yellow colour, found in foods like squashes and fizzy drinks, marzipan and piccalilli sauce.

E104 Quinoline yellow
A dull yellow coloured azo dye found in smoked haddock and Scotch eggs.

E110 Sunset yellow FCF; Orange yellow S
A yellow azo dye added to packets of breadcrumbs and apricot jam, packet soups and sweets.

E120 Cochineal; Carminic acid; Carmines
A natural colour from the egg yolks and dried parts of a female beetle which lives in countries in Central America and the West Indies. 70,000 insects are needed to produce 1lb of colour. It is very expensive and so not often used these days in food manufacturing.

E122 Azorubine; Carmoisine
A synthetic azo dye with a red colour, which is found in blancmanges and sweets, packet jellies and Swiss rolls.

E123 Amaranth
A red azo colour found in tinned fruit pie fillings, packets of cake, soup and trifle mixes and gravy granules.

E124 Ponceau 4R; Cochineal red A
Often used instead of 'real' cochineal, this synthetic azo dye has a red colour and is found in canned strawberries and cherries, canned raspberry pie fillings, packets of soup and cake, and quick-set jelly mixes.

E127 Erythrosine
A red azo in colour and found in Scotch eggs and glacé cherries, biscuits and canned strawberries and rhubarb.

E128 Red 2G
A red azo colour used in sausages and cooked meat products like burgers.

E129 Allura red AC
A red azo dye used in sweet drinks and condiments.

E131 Patent blue V
A deep violet-blue-coloured azo dye. It is not widely used but is found in Scotch eggs.

E132 Indigotine; Indigo carmine
A blue azo colour used in biscuits, sweets and blancmange.

E133 Brilliant blue FCF
A synthetic azo dye that gives a blue colour, but with tones of green if used with a yellow colouring. Found in canned peas.

E140 Chlorophyll and Chlorophyllins
Cholorophyll is the natural green pigment in plants. When used as a colouring agent it is usually mixed with other plant pigments. It is used in oils and naturally green vegetables and fruits stored in liquids.

E141 Copper complexes of chlorophyll and chlorophyllins
This colour is derived from chlorophyll. The copper complexes of chlorophyll have an olive-green colour and the chlorophyllins have a straight green colour. Used in vegetables and fruits preserved in water.

E142 Green S

A green azo dye used in canned peas, gravy granules and mint sauces and jellies.

E150a Plain caramel
E150b Caustic sulphite caramel
E150c Ammonia caramel
E150d Sulphite ammonia caramel

Caramels are produced through heating carbohydrates to give a brown colour. They also impart a caramel flavour and can be found in foods like biscuits and pickled onions, gravy mixes, soya sauce and fruit sauce. These caramel colourings are the most frequently used group, making up 98 per cent of all colourings used in foods and drinks.

E151 Brilliant black BN; Black PN

A synthetic black azo dye used in the colouring of blackcurrant cheesecake mixes and brown sauces.

E153 Vegetable carbon

This black colour simply comes from burning plant material and is used in jams and jellies.

E154 Brown FK

A synthetic azo dye mix giving foods like kippers and smoked mackerel a brown colour.

E155 Brown HT

A brown azo dye found mainly in chocolate-flavoured cakes.

E160a Carotenes

These are extracts from plants like carrots and tomatoes, oranges and green leafy vegetables such as spinach. Carotenes have a yellowy-orange colour and are found in spreadable margarine, yoghurts and foods like sponge cakes.

E160b Annatto; Bixin; Norbixin
This vegetable dye comes from the seeds of the Annatto tree, which grows in the Tropics and has a peachy yellow colour. It is found in anything from Cheshire cheese and butter to tubs of coleslaw and sponge puddings.

E160c Paprika extract; Capsanthian; Capsorubin
Naturally produced from the red spice paprika, the orange colour that is extracted is used in foods like processed cheese slices.

E160d Lycopene
The vibrant red pigment extracted from tomatoes, lycopene is added to give a red colour to foods.

E160e Beta–apo–8'–carotenal (C30)
This natural yellow colour is again extracted from plants and gives a yellow-orange colour to foods.

E160f Ethyl ester of beta–apo–8'–carotenoic acid (C30)
A plant extract with a natural yellow-to-orange pigment.

E161b Lutein
Lutein has a yellow colour and is derived from green-leafed plants like spinach.

E161g Canthaxanthin
This carotene is found in mushrooms and has a natural orange colour. It is used in foods like marshmallow biscuits.

E162 Beetroot red; Betanin
The deep purple natural food colouring is the pigment extracted from beetroot. It is used in foods like oxtail soup.

E163 Anthocyanins
These blue, violet or red pigments are natural colours extracted from berries, stems and leaves of plants.

E170 Calcium carbonate
This is simply the scientific name for chalk, which is used as an acidity regulator in wine to lower the pH. This naturally occurring mineral has a white colour and is used in biscuits and buns, cakes, ice cream, sweets and bread.

E171 Titanium dioxide
Made from the natural mineral ilmenite, it gives a white colour to foods and is used in products such as cottage cheese, and horseradish creams and sauces.

E172 Iron oxides and hydroxides
These naturally-occurring red, brown, black, orange and yellow colours are used to give colour to cake and dessert mixes and to salmon and shrimp pastes.

E173 Aluminium
Another naturally-occurring colouring used on the surface of foods like sugar-coated cake decorations to give a metallic look.

E174 Silver
A naturally-occurring mineral used on the surface of cake decorations to give a metallic colour.

E175 Gold
A naturally-occurring mineral to give a gold metallic look to cake decorations, again, only to be used on their surface.

E180 Litholrubine BK
A synthetic azo dye with a red colour that is used to colour the rind of cheese.

Preservatives
E200 Sorbic acid
This can be extracted naturally from berries and be synthetically produced. It is added to foods to stop the growth of yeast and moulds and is found in yoghurts and sweets, soft drinks and processed cheese slices, as well as frozen pizzas and ready-made cakes. Wine and cider, dessert sauces and candied peel can also contain sorbic acid.

E202 Potassium sorbate
A synthetic preservative used for its antibacterial and anti-fungal properties in foods like salad and seafood dressings, ready-made cakes, frozen pizzas and margarine.

E203 Calcium sorbate
A synthetic preservative with antibacterial and anti-fungal properties, found in yoghurts and fermented milks.

E210 Benzoic acid
Benzoic acid is found naturally in berries but is synthetically produced as a food preservative. It is used for its antibacterial and anti-fungal properties in everything from beer and fruit juice to coffee essence and marinated herrings.

E211 Sodium benzoate
A preservative made from benzoic acid with an anti-bacterial and

anti-fungal activity that works when a food is slightly acidic. For this reason it is found in products like soya, oyster sauce and orange squash plus prawns, sweets and even caviar.

E212 Potassium benzoate
A preservative also made from benzoic acid with anti-bacterial and anti-fungal properties.

E213 Calcium benzoate
Another preservative derived from benzoic acid with an anti-bacterial and anti-fungal activity.

E214 Ethyl p-hydroxybenzoate
A preservative again made from benzoic acid with an anti-bacterial and anti-fungal activity. Found in foods like marinated herrings and mackerel, fruit pie fillings, cooked beetroot, salad creams and jams.

E215 Sodium ethyl p-hydroxybenzoate
Guess what? Another benzoic acid-derived preservative with anti-bacterial and anti-fungal properties.

E216 Propyl p-hydroxybenzoate
And again. An anti-microbial preservative made from benzoic acid found in beer and fruit purées, pickles and salad creams, among other products.

E217 Sodium propyl p-hydroxybenzoate
And finally, the last anti-microbial preservative based on benzoic acid.

E218 Methyl p-hydroxybenzoate
This synthetic preservative is an anti-microbial found, for instance, in beer and flavoured syrups, pickles and salad creams, snack meals and dessert sauces.

E219 Sodium methyl p-hydroxybenzoate
Back to benzoic acid: this derivative has anti-fungal and anti-yeast activity.

E220 Sulphur dioxide
This preservative occurs naturally but is produced by a chemical process to create an additive for the food industry that has preserving qualities. It is used in foods such as packet soups and fruit juices, dry root ginger, canned crab meat and sausage meat, to mention just a handful. This preservative also has antioxidant properties and is permitted in wine- and cider-making to rid the drinks of microbes that could otherwise set up infections, and to prevent discolouration.

E221 Sodium sulphite
A synthetic preservative with anti-microbial activity used to help preserve egg yolk.

E222 Sodium hydrogen sulphite
A synthetic preservative.

E223 Sodium metabisulphite
A synthetic preservative used in orange squash, pickled onions and red cabbage. It is also found in packets of mashed potatoes and tubs of salads.

E224 Potassium metabisulphite
A synthetic preservative found in Campden Tablets. Used for making home-made wine.

E226 Calcium sulphite
A synthetic preservative used in cider.

E227 Calcium hydrogen sulphite
A synthetic preservative used in beer.

E228 Potassium hydrogen sulphite
A synthetic preservative.

E230 Biphenyl; Diphenyl
A synthetic preservative with anti-fungal properties used in treating lemon, orange and grapefruit skins. It can be partially removed by washing off with detergents.

E231 Orthophenyl phenol
A synthetic antibacterial and anti-fungal preservative found on the skins of oranges, lemons and other citrus fruit like grapefruit.

E232 Sodium orthophenyl phenol
A synthetic preservative used for its anti-fungal properties on the surface of citrus fruit.

E234 Nisin
A preservative made from a Streptococcus bacterium used in cottage cheese, cheese and clotted cream. It is also found in some canned foods.

E235 Natamycin
Protects cheese from mould and yeast growth.

E239 Hexamethylene tetramine
A synthetic preservative which is anti-fungal and can be found in marinated herrings.

E249 Potassium nitrite
A naturally-occurring preservative used in cooked meats and sausages.

E250 Sodium nitrite
A man-made anti-bacterial preservative used in sausages, bacon, ham and tongue; pressed, cured and canned meats; smoked frankfurters and, among other foods, frozen pizza. It is used in the curing of ham and bacon to give it a reddish colour.

E251 Sodium nitrate
A mineral that occurs naturally and is used in bacon and ham, beef, canned meats, tongue and frozen pizza. These minerals are naturally mined and can be used just in curing ham and bacon.

E252 Potassium nitrate
Potassium nitrate occurs naturally and can be made to preserve foods such as cured meats, sausages, canned meats, bacon and ham.

E280 Propionic acid
A type of fatty acid found naturally which has anti-fungal activity. It is used in pizzas and baked products as well as dairy foods.

E281 Sodium propionate
Derived from propionic acid, this preservative fights fungi and is found in baked and dairy foods.

E282 Calcium propionate
While calcium propionate is found naturally in some cheeses, it is manufactured commercially for use as a preservative. Able to inhibit mould, it is used in baked products, dairy foods and frozen pizza.

E283 Potassium propionate
Made from propionic acid, this preservative inhibits the growth of mould and is found in Christmas puddings as well as baked and dairy products.

E284 Boric acid
An acidity regulator.

E285 Sodium tetraborate; Borax
Also an acidity regulator used on, rather than in, foods as an inorganic herbicide.

E1105 Lysozyme
An enzyme naturally found in egg white and bodily fluids which acts as a mild antiseptic. It is made from egg albumen and kills bacteria.

Antioxidants
E300 Ascorbic acid
Also known as vitamin C, this antioxidant can be the 'real' thing or a synthetic version. It is used in flour, beer, jam and fruit drink concentrates.

E301 Sodium ascorbate
A synthetic antioxidant, this is found in foods like Scotch eggs and sausages.

E302 Calcium ascorbate
A synthetic antioxidant used in Scotch eggs.

E304 Fatty acid esters of ascorbic acid
A synthetic antioxidant used in Scotch eggs, sausages and some stock cubes.

E306 Tocopherol
This is natural vitamin E derived from vegetable oils. It is then added to other vegetable oils to top up levels and help stop them from going rancid.

E307 Alpha-tocopherol
A synthetic version of vitamin E used in sausages.

E308 Gamma-tocopherol
Another synthetic version of vitamin E.

E309 Delta-tocopherol
Again, a synthetic version of vitamin E.

E310 Propyl gallate
A synthetically-made antioxidant used in chewing gum, snack foods, vegetable oils and margarine.

E311 Octyl gallate
A synthetic antioxidant used in oils, margarine and salad dressings.

E312 Dodecyl gallate
A synthetic antioxidant used in oils, margarine and salad dressings.

E320 Butylated hydroxyanisole (BHA)
A synthetically-made antioxidant found in lots of foods, including biscuits and butter, cheese spreads and margarine, fruit pies, soft drinks and stock cubes.

E321 Butylated hydroxytoluene (BHT)
A synthetic antioxidant used in chewing gum and peanuts, gravy granules, cake mixes, crisps and even breakfast cereals.

Sweeteners
E420
(i) Sorbitol
Sorbitol is a type of bulk sugar alcohol found naturally in cherries,

apricots, plums and apples. It is made from the fruit sugar fructose. Digestion of its calories in the digestive system is very slow. It is found in foods like reduced-sugar jam and foods designed for people with diabetes. Sorbitol supplies 4 calories per gram.

(ii) Sorbitol syrup
A syrup version of sorbitol.

E421 Mannitol
Also called manna sugar, mannitol is found in beetroot, pumpkin, mushrooms and onion, but is made commercially from the seaweed Laminaria. Found in sugar-free sweets, it is about 60 per cent as sweet as sugar (sucrose). Mannitol supplies 4 calories per gram.

E953 Isomalt
A bulk sweetener which is about half as sweet as sugar (sucrose). Used in 'Tooth Friendly' sugar-free sweets, it supplies 4 calories per gram.

E965
(i) Maltitol
A so-called 'polyol' sugar alcohol sweetener made from the naturally-occurring sugar maltose. It is digested slowly and broken down into sorbitol and glucose in the intestine. It is about 10 per cent less sweet than sugar and is found in sugar-free sweets. It supplies 4 calories per gram.

(ii) Maltitol syrup
A syrup version of maltitol.

E966 Lactitol
This sugar alcohol is made from lactulose, a type of carbohydrate formed when milk is heated. It is not digested by enzymes in the intestinal tract but moves into the colon where it is fermented by

bacteria. Unlike sugar (sucrose) and most other bulk sweeteners that supply 4 calories per gram, lactitol provides just 2 calories per gram. It is less sweet than sugar.

E967 Xylitol

Xylitol occurs naturally in raspberries, endive, lettuce and in the wood of the birch tree, which is the source of commercial xylitol. It is a sugar alcohol, which is about 80 per cent as sweet as sugar. It helps to inhibit the growth of bacteria that cause tooth decay and is used in sugar-free sweets and sugar-free chewing gum. Xylitol supplies 4 calories per gram.

E950 Acesulfame K

A synthetic intense sweetener made from a chemical called 'oxathiazinone'. Acesulfame K is the potassium salt of this chemical and is 200 times sweeter than sugar (sucrose). It is calorie-free and moves through the body undigested.

E951 Aspartame

This artificial sweetener is made from two protein building blocks that occur naturally in foods, called aspartic acid and phenylalanine. It is 200 times sweeter than sugar (sucrose) and is used in fizzy drinks, tabletop sweeteners and dessert mixes. Aspartame is calorie-free.

E952 Cyclamic acid and its Na and Ca salts

Thirty times sweeter than sugar (sucrose), cyclamate can be heated (unlike saccharin) and can be used in baked foods.

E954 Saccharin and its Na, K and Ca salts

Five hundred and fifty times sweeter than sugar (sucrose), saccharin is a synthetic sweetener made from benzoic sulphimide. It is calorie-free and found in sugar-free sweets and drinks, and foods designed for people with diabetes.

E957 Thaumatin
An astonishing 1,600 times sweeter than sugar, thaumatin is an incredibly sweet protein found in the African fruit Thaumatococcus danielli. Called 'katemfe' in Sierra Leone and a 'miracle fruit' in the Sudan, it is calorie-free.

E959 Neohesperidine DC
Another very intense sweeter, 1,000 times sweeter than sugar (sucrose), this is formed from the naturally-occurring supernutrient neohesperidin, found in citrus fruit.

Sucralose
The trade name of the intense sweetener, this is 2,000 times sweeter than sugar (sucrose) and is made from chlorinated sucrose. No E number has been given to sucralose yet as it has not been fully authorized across the EU.

Permitted sweeteners may not be used in or on any infant foods intended for children under 12 months, or for young children between one and three years of age.

Emulsifiers, stabilizers, thickeners and gelling agents
E322 Lecithins
Lecithins are naturally present in egg yolk and soya beans, both of which are commercial sources of this additive. Lecithins are added to food for their properties, which include emulsifying, stabilizing and antioxidant activity. They are used in foods such as chocolate and sweets, margarines, powdered milks and dessert mixes.

E400 Alginic acid
This additive is extracted from Laminaria, which are brown seaweeds. It is used as a thickener, gelling agent, stabilizer and emulsifier. Alginic acid is found in foods like ice cream, puddings and instant dessert mixes.

E401 Sodium alginate

This additive is made from alginic acid and is used for its stabilizing effects as well as its ability to suspend, thicken and emulsify. It can be found in puddings and ice cream, barbecue sauce mixes and canned fruit fillings.

E402 Potassium alginate

Another derivative of alginic acid, potassium alginate can help foods to gel as well as acting as a stabilizing and emulsifying agent.

E403 Ammonium alginate

Again, prepared from alginic acid, this is used to thicken, stabilize and emulsify.

E404 Calcium alginate

Another alginic acid derivative, this emulsifier, stabilizer, thickener and gelling agent is used in synthetic cream and ice cream.

E405 Propane-1,2-diol alginate

The final alginic acid derivative, as well as having emulsifying, stabilizing and thickening properties, it acts as a solvent for carrying spices. It is found in mint sauces and seafood dressing, as well as foods like cottage cheese that contains salmon, and Thousand Island dressing.

E406 Agar

Naturally occurring in the stems of red seaweed like *Gelidium amansi*, agar is a thickening and gelling agent that also has stabilizing properties. It is used to thicken ice cream and can be found in frozen trifle and some meat products.

E407 Carrageenan

Carrageenan comes from seaweeds such as *Chondrus crispus*. It helps to emulsify, thicken and gel and is found in a wide variety of foods such as blancmanges and frozen trifles; cheese and sour cream; pastries and biscuits; milk shakes; canned whipped cream and alcoholic drinks. It is also allowed in infant foods.

E407a Processed eucheuma seaweed
A processed version of a seaweed extract.

E410 Locust bean gum; Carob gum
This gelling, stabilizing and emulsifying agent is derived from the seeds of the Carob, which is also known as the Locust tree. A member of the pea family, it is used in things like coleslaw and Italian ice cream.

E412 Guar gum
Guar gum comes from the seeds of plants that belong to the pea family called *Cyamopis tetragonolobus*. It adds bulk to foods, thickens, emulsifies and stabilizes food. Among other products, it is added to brown sauce and piccalilli, frozen fruits, fruit drinks, ice cream and milkshakes.

E413 Tragacanth
This is a gum extracted from the branches of the bush called *Astragalus gummifer*, which is also a member of the pea family. It helps to stop sugar from crystallizing in sweets, and emulsifies, stabilizes and thickens foods like cottage cheese with added salmon, salad dressings and cream cheese. It is also found in cake decorations and sherbet.

E414 Acacia gum; Gum arabic
This gum comes from the African acacia tree, a member of the pea family. The gum thickens, stabilizes and emulsifies and acts as a glazing agent. It helps to stop sugar from crystallizing.

E415 Xanthan gum
This gum is actually produced by carbohydrate fermentation. It stabilizes, thickens and emulsifies and is used in products like seafood dressings and frozen pizza, canned fruit pie fillings and coleslaw.

E416 Karaya gum
A gum which comes from trees native to China, called the *Sterculiaceae* family. It is able to stabilize, emulsify and thicken foods and is found in certain cheeses, brown sauces and piccalilli.

E417 Tara gum
From the seeds of the tara gum tree, it has the gelling properties of agar.

E418 Gellan gum
A complex carbohydrate produced by fermentation, this gel is used in certain fruit drinks.

E425 Konjac
Konjac gum comes from the tubers of the *Amorphophallus konjac* plant, grown in Japan.

E432 Polyoxyethylene sorbitan monolaurate; Polysorbate 20
This emulsifier and stabilizer is made from sorbitol. It is used to improve the volume and texture in baked goods.

E433 Polyoxyethylene sorbitan mono-oleate; Polysorbate 80
Like E432, this emulsifier and stabilizer is prepared from sorbitol. It is used to improve the volume and texture in baked goods.

E434 Polyoxyethylene sorbitan monopalmitate; Polysorbate 40
Again prepared from sorbitol, this additive emulsifies and stabilizes and is used in desserts and sugar confectionery.

E435 Polyoxyethylene sorbitan monostearate; Polysorbate 60
Another derivative of sorbitol, this emulsifier and stabilizer is found in cake mixes.

E436 Polyoxyethylene sorbitan tristearate; Polysorbate 65
This additive is an emulsifier and stabilizer made from sorbitol.

E440 Pectin
Pectin comes from the spaces between the cell walls of plants. It acts as an emulsifier and can help to form a gel in an acid environment, such as jam and fruit jelly. It is also found in marmalade, puddings and cold desserts.

E442 Ammonium phosphatides
Made from pectin, this additive acts as a stabilizing and gelling agent and has thickening properties. It is found in jellies and jam.

E444 Sucrose acetate isobutyrate
Derived from cane sugar.

E445 Glycerol esters of wood resins
This is extracted from wood pulp and used in some soft drinks

E460 Cellulose
Cellulose comes from the cell walls of plants and is used as a bulking and anti-caking agent and for its ability to bind, thicken, filter and disperse.

E461 Methyl cellulose
E463 Hydroxypropyl cellulose
E464 Hydroxypropyl methyl cellulose
E465 Ethyl methyl cellulose
Made from cellulose, these additives act as a foaming agent as well as having emulsifying and stabilizing effects in food.

E466 Carboxy methyl cellulose; Sodium carboxy methyl cellulose
Created chemically, this additive has the ability to thicken, modify textures, act as a stabilizer, keep moisture under control, gel, bulk and create an opaque effect in foods. It is found in a wide variety of foods from meringues and ice cream to tomato sauces and frozen chips; diet squashes; and processed and cottage cheeses.

E470a Sodium, potassium and calcium salts of fatty acids
E470b Magnesium salts of fatty acids
Both of these additives are prepared chemically and act as anti-caking, emulsifying and stabilizing agents. Found in foods like savoury snacks, crisps and packets of pudding mixes.

E471 Mono- and diglycerides of fatty acids
This additive is made from glycerin and fatty acids and is found in foods like ready-made cakes and aerosol cream, hot chocolate drink mixes and quick custard powder mixes.

E472a Acetic acid esters of mono- and diglycerides of fatty acids
Made from acetic acid (vinegar) it helps to emulsify, stabilize and modify the texture of foods. It is also known for its ability to act as a solvent and lubricant and is found in packets of cheesecake and other dessert mixes.

E472b Lactic acid esters of mono- and diglycerides of fatty acids
Made from lactic acid (the acid in soured milk), this has emulsifying and stabilizing properties and is found in dessert mixes.

E472c Citric acid esters of mono- and diglycerides of fatty acids
Made from the citric acid found in citrus fruits, this additive emulsifies and stabilizes and is found in packet desserts.

E472d Tartaric acid esters of mono- and diglycerides of fatty acids
This emulsifier and stabiliser is made from tartaric acid found naturally in grapes and is added to packet dessert toppings.

E472e Mono- and diacetyltartaric acid esters of mono- and diglycerides of fatty acids
Made from tartaric acid, this emulsifiying and stabilizing additive is found in brown bread rolls, frozen pizza, gravy granules and hot chocolate powder.

E472f Mixed acetic and tartaric acid esters of mono- and diglycerides of fatty acids
A dough conditioner in yeast-raised bakery products, hot chocolate mixes, pizzas and gravy granules.

E473 Sucrose esters of fatty acids
Made from fatty acids, this emulsifier and stabilizer is used in margarines, mayonnaise soups and dairy desserts.

E474 Sucroglycerides
This emulsifier and stabilizer is made from sucrose acting on triglycerides. It is found in lard and palm oil and used in dairy-based drinks, coffee whiteners and dairy-based desserts.

E475 Polyglycerol esters of fatty acids
A synthetically created emulsifier and stabilizer, this additive is found in packets of cheesecake and cake mixes and ready-made sponges and cakes.

E476 Polyglycerol polyricinoleate
Made from castor oil, this is a stabilizer and emulsifier used in icing toppings and cake mixes.

E477 Propane-1,2-diol esters of fatty acids
A man-made emulsifier and stabilizer, this can be found in packets of cake and instant dessert mixes.

E479b Thermally oxidized soya-bean oil interacted with mono- and diglycerides of fatty acids
This is used in margarine.

E481 Sodium stearoyl-2-lactylate
Made from lactic acid, the acid formed in soured milk, this stabilizer and emulsifier is found in cakes, bread and biscuits.

E482 Calcium stearoyl-2-lactylate
Made synthetically, this is used as a whipping agent as well as for its stabilizing and emulsifying properties. It is found in gravy granules.

E483 Stearyl tartrate
Made from tartaric acid found in grapes, this additive is a stabilizer and emulsifier. A dough-strengthening agent.

E491 Sorbitan monostearate
Used for its ability to give foods a glaze, E491 is made from stearic acid. It is found in most animal and vegetable fats. It also acts as an emulsifier and stabilizer and is added to packet cake mixes.

E492 Sorbitan tristearate
Made from stearic acid found in vegetable oils, this is an emulsifier and stabilizer.

E493 Sorbitan monolaurate
Made from lauric acid found in butter, palm and coconut oil, E493 has antifoaming abilities as well as acting as an emulsifier and stabilizer.

E494 Sorbitan mono-oleate
Made from oleic acid found in olive and rapeseed oil, this additive stabilizes and emulsifies.

E495 Sorbitan monopalmitate
Chemically created, this emulsifier is soluble in oil and acts as a stabilizer in foods.

E1103 Invertase
Invertase is an enzyme that splits sugar (sucrose) into glucose and fructose. Also known as sucrase and saccharase. Used in confectionery and in the liquid and soft centres of chocolates.

'Others'
In addition to these main groups of additives, there is a miscellaneous group known as 'others'. They function as acidity regulators, anti-caking agents, anti-foaming agents, bulking agents, firming agents, flavour enhancers, foaming agents, humectants, modified starches, packaging gases, propellants, raising agents, carrier solvents, emulsifying salts, acids and sequestrants.

E170 Calcium carbonates
Also known simply as 'chalk', this naturally-occurring mineral has various roles in food processing. For instance, it acts as an alkali to balance up pH levels, it gives firmness to foods, can act as a releasing agent in vitamin tablets, is used to colour the surface of foods, and is found in calcium supplements.

E260 Acetic acid
This is the acid of vinegar and is formed naturally. It has antibacterial functions and is also added to food to stabilize acidity and dilute colouring. It is found in salad creams, brown sauces, pickles, chutneys,

cheese, and in mint and other sauces.

E261 Potassium acetate
An additive which is used to maintain the natural colour of plant and animal tissues to stop them fading. Technically, it is the potassium salt of acetic acid.

E262 Sodium acetate
This is the sodium salt of acetic acid and is used to buffer a food or drink's acidic or alkaline nature.

E263 Calcium acetate
The calcium salt of acetic acid, calcium acetate has several roles including an ability to firm foods, prevent the growth of mould, and act as a preservative and a sequestrant.

E270 Lactic acid
Lactic acid is produced by the fermentation of carbohydrates and was originally discovered in soured milk. It gives the flavour to fermented milk. It is able to suppress bacterial growth and is added to foods for its preservative effects, its ability to increase the anti-oxidant effect of other substances, and to give acidity and flavouring. It is used in sweets, soft drinks, pickles, sauces and pickled red cabbage.

E290 Carbon dioxide
A gas present in our atmosphere, this is used for its preservative effects, as a packaging gas, to cool products and to freeze foods when in its liquid form. It is found, for example, in mineral water and fizzy drinks.

E296 Malic acid
An acid that naturally occurs in lots of fruits, especially apples, tomatoes and plums, this is a food additive that is used to increase the

acidity of foods like tinned soups, and drinks such as low-calorie orange squash. Malic acid is used in cider to lower the pH and so increase acidity.

E297 Fumaric acid
Found in packet desserts and bakery goods, this natural 'organic' acid acts as a flavouring and is used to help foods rise. It also has an anti-oxidant role when used in cakes.

E325 Sodium lactate
This additive is technically known as the sodium salt of the other additive, lactic acid. It increases the anti-oxidant effect in foods and has the ability to absorb moisture in its role as a humectant. It can be found in sweets and cheese.

E326 Potassium lactate
The potassium salt of lactic acid, this acts as a buffer in foods. Like sodium lactate, it increases the anti-oxidant levels of foods.

E327 Calcium lactate
The calcium salt of lactic acid, it has an ability to add firmness to foods, acts as a buffer and has an anti-oxidant role. Calcium lactate can be found in dessert mixes.

E330 Citric acid
What is known as an 'organic' acid, citric acid is found widely in foods throughout nature, especially lemons. For its use in food processing it is made by fermenting the mould *Aspergillus niger* or is simply taken from citrus fruits. It is used as a flavouring and acidifying agent. Citric acid is used widely and can be found in everything from ice cream and jam to frozen fish, cheese and cakes, as well as in the treatment of dried fruits.

E331 Sodium citrates
A salt of citric acid, sodium citrate is able to help regulate and buffer the acidity of foods and acts as an emulsifier. It is found in confectionery, packet puddings and sometimes ice cream.

E332 Potassium citrates
This is another salt of citric acid and, like sodium citrate, regulates acidity and acts as an emulsifier. It is found, for example, in dried and condensed milk, and cheese.

E333 Calcium citrates
The calcium salt of citric acid, not only does calcium citrate help emulsify ingredients in food, it also buffers acidity and alkalinity as well as having an ability to help firm foods. It is found in sweets, fizzy drinks and some cheeses.

E334 Tartaric acid
Tartaric acid is found naturally in fruits, especially grapes. It is added to lemonade and jams to increase their acidity and is also found in baking powder. It can increase the anti-oxidant level in foods, has sequestrant roles in food processing, and is used to dilute food colourings before they are added to foods and fizzy drinks.

E335 Sodium tartrates
Sodium tartrates are made from tartaric acid and are found naturally in grapes, as well as in foods like marmalade and jams, fizzy drinks and sweets. They act as buffers, raising the anti-oxidant level of a food and have both sequestrant and emulsifying roles in food processing.

E336 Potassium tartrates
Known to cooks simply as 'cream of tartare', one of its most familiar uses is as a raising agent in flour. It is also added to foods like packet desserts to give acidity and act as an emulsifier.

E337 Sodium potassium tartrate
Also known as Rochelle salt, this additive is found in cheese and meat products. As well as acting as a stabilizing agent, it has the ability to increase the anti-oxidant levels in foods. It has an emulsifying capacity and can also buffer the acidity and alkalinity of products.

E338–E343
E338 phosphoric acid and its salts; E339 sodium phosphates; E340 potassium phosphates; E341 calcium phosphates and E343 magnesium phosphates. These are used to regulate acidity in acid fruit-flavoured drinks like lemonade. They are also found in foods like ham and sausages, cheese and pudding mixes.

E341 (A) Monocalcium phosphate
This is used as a raising agent in self-raising flours and comes from the mineral apartite.

E350–352
These are all sodium malates. Malic acid is a naturally-occurring acid found in lots of fruits including apples, tomatoes and plums. E350 sodium malate, E351 potassium malate and E352 Calcium malate are salts of malic acid and are used in foods to increase the acidity levels and to act as buffers.

E353 Metatartaric acid
Found in wine, this is made from tartaric acid and is added to food for its sequestrant properties.

E354 Calcium tartrate
Used in biscuits and rusks.

E355 Adipic acid
While adipic acid is found naturally in some plants, it is also manufactured synthetically for use in food processing where it has the ability to increase the acidity of food. It is used to increase acidic flavours and as a raising agent in baking powder.

E356–E357
Both sodium adipates, these are derived from adipic acid and have similar roles in food processing.

E363 Succinic acid
Produced synthetically for food processing, succinic acid can be found in nature but only occurs in odd places like fungi. It is manufactured for its acid-enhancing role in food processing and as a flavour enhancer.

E380 Triammonium citrate
An additive that is made from citric acid, this is used for its ability to buffer foods and to act as an emulsifying salt.

E385 Calcium disodium ethylene diamine tetra-acetate; Calcium disodium EDTA
Also known as versene, sequestrol and sequestrene, this additive is found in foods like dressings for salads. It has the ability to bind trace metals found in food, like copper, which makes it a chelating agent, and it also has a sequestrant role.

E391 Nitrogen (also E941)
A natural gas used in the packaging of foods like pre-packed salads, to extend their shelf life.

E422 Glycerol
Glycerol is a colourless, sticky liquid that is sweet to taste. It is made

from fats and used in foods as a humectant to help keep them moist, in cakes and batters to improve texture and slow down the staling process, and to dissolve flavourings.

E431 Polyoxyethylene (40) stearate
Made from fats, this emulsifier is added to bread to give it a softer crumb and to slow down staling.

E450 Diphosphates
Made synthetically, this additive can be found in dried and condensed milk, whipping cream and cheese. It is used for its ability to gel, emulsify, stabilize and buffer the acidity and alkalinity of foods.

E451–E452
E451 triphosphates and E452 polyphosphates are found, among other foods, in cheeses and sausages where they act as emulsifiers and give texture to foods.

E459 Beta–cyclodextrin
A glazing agent restricted to foods in tablet and coated tablet form, and as a carrier solvent for other additives.

E500–E504
E500 Sodium carbonates, E501 Potassium carbonates, E503 Ammonium carbonates and E504 Magnesium carbonates are made synthetically and act as buffers and neutralizers in foods. They are found, for example, in baking and custard powder. E503 is a raising agent used in bakery products, made by mixing ammonium sulphate with chalk.

E507 Hydrochloric acid
This acid is found naturally in our stomachs where it helps to digest protein and beat the bacteria we eat in foods and drinks. In food

processing a synthetic version is used which is added to increase acidity.

E508 Potassium chloride
A natural salt, potassium chloride is used in salt substitute products. It is also used as a stabilizer and emulsifier in foods. E508 is found in low sodium and low salt foods.

E509 Calcium chloride
A naturally prepared additive, calcium chloride can be found in canned pulses, like red kidney beans, to which it is added to give firmness. It is also a sequestrant. It is used in soy-bean curd (tofu) to help the soy milk coagulate during processing. It comes from natural salt brines.

E511 Magnesium chloride
A colour retention agent generally permitted for use as an additive in most processed foods – also used as a source of magnesium in fortified products.

E512 Stannous chloride
A colour stabilizer restricted to canned and bottled foods and white asparagus.

E513 Sulphuric acid
Very small amounts are used in food processing to increase the acidity of a food.

E514 Sodium sulphates
Used in food processing to dilute products.

E515 Potassium sulphates
Used in food processing as a substitute for salt.

E516 Calcium sulphate

This natural mineral is also known as gypsum and is used to carry vitamins and minerals that are added to foods like flour. It is also used as a coagulation additive in soy-bean curd. It has a range of roles as an additive including the ability to act as a firming agent and a sequestrant. It is also used in the fortification of food, as a nutrient to increase the calcium content of a food.

E517 Ammonium sulphate

An acidity regulator and firming agent. Permitted for use as a carrier solvent.

E520 Aluminium sulphate
E521 Aluminium sodium sulphate
E522 Aluminium potassium sulphate
E523 Aluminium ammonium sulphate

These are stabilizers and permitted use is restricted to egg white and candied, crystallized and glazed fruit and vegetables.

E524 Sodium hydroxide

Found in jam, this additive is used to dissolve colours in.

E525 Potassium hydroxide

Used as a base in cocoa products, potassium hydroxide is made synthetically.

E526 Calcium hydroxide

Made from lime, calcium hydroxide helps to firm foods and is used as a neutralizing agent. It is used in foods like cocoa products and cheese, plus some crisps.

E527 Ammonium hydroxide
Used to dilute colours, E527 is also an alkali and is found in food-colouring preparations and in cocoa products.

E528 Magnesium hydroxide
Found in cocoa products, this additive is used for its alkali properties.

E529 Calcium oxide
Used to increase the calcium content of foods, this is also an alkali and is found in various cocoa products.

E530 Magnesium oxide
A natural rock mineral, this additive is used for its anti-caking properties and for its alkali nature to help the processing of cocoa products.

E535, E536, E538
All prepared synthetically, E535 Sodium ferrocyanide, E536 Potassium ferrocyanide and E538 Calcium ferrocyanide have anti-caking properties.

E541 Sodium aluminium phosphate
A synthetically prepared additive, it is found in cake mixes for its raising properties. It also increases acidity of foods.

E551 Silicon dioxide
Also known as silica or silicea, this is a mineral used to help thicken foods and also for its anti-caking and stabilizing properties. It can be found in wine and crisps.

E552–E570
E552 Calcium silicate; E553a (i) Magnesium silicate, (ii) Magnesium trisilicate; E553b Talc; E554 Sodium aluminium silicate; E555

Potassium aluminium silicate; E556 Aluminium calcium silicate; E558 Bentonite; E559 Aluminium silicate; and E570 Kaolin. These fatty acids all have anti-caking properties and can be found in foods like packet cake mixes, sweets and noodles.

E574 Gluconic acid
This acid is made synthetically. It is also known as dextronic, maltonic and glycogenic acid and is added to foods for its ability to increase acidity.

E575–E579
E575 Glucono delta-lactone; E576 Sodium gluconate; E577 Potassium gluconate; E578 Calcium gluconate and E579 Ferrous gluconate all act as sequestrants and can be found in foods like packet cake mixes.

E585 Ferrous lactate
A colour stabilizer restricted to olives darkened by oxidation.

E620 Glutamic acid
A protein building block known as an 'amino acid', glutamic acid is used as a flavour enhancer and to replace salt in foods.

E621 Monosodium glutamate
Known simply as MSG, glutamate occurs naturally in sundried tomatoes, Parmesan cheese and Setango seaweed. MSG is the sodium salt of glutamic acid and is prepared synthetically and used in many foods, from soups and flavoured noodles to canned meats.

E622–E635
E622 Monopotassium glutamate; E623 Calcium diglutamate; E624 Monoammonium glutamate; E625 Magnesium diglutamate; E626 Guanylic acid; E627 Disodium guanylate; E628 Dipotassium guanylate; E629 Calcium guanylate; E630 Inosinic acid; E631 Disodium inosinate;

E632 Dipotassium inosinate; E633 Calcium inosinate; E634 Calcium 5'-ribonucleotides, and E635 Disodium 5'-ribonucleotides. These are all synthetically prepared flavour enhancers. Typically, they can be found in foods like crisps and gravy granules, potato waffles and pre-cooked dried rice snacks.

E640 Glycine and its sodium salt
A preservative used as an anti-oxidant and flavour enhancer, generally permitted for use in most processed foods.

E650 Zinc acetate
A flavour enhancer. Permitted use is restricted to chewing gum.

E900 Dimethylpolysiloxane
A synthetic anti-foaming agent made from silica gel or silicon dioxide with a liquid called dimethylpolysiloxane. It is found in foods such as jam.

E901 Beeswax, white and yellow
Used to help give foods a polished, glazed look, this natural additive comes from the honeycomb of bees.

E902 Candelilla wax
An anti-caking and glazing agent used in confectionery, chocolate-coated fine bakery, snacks, nuts, coffee beans, dietary food supplements, fresh citrus fruit, melons, apples, pears, peaches and pineapples.

E903 Carnauba wax
This wax comes from the leaves of a Brazilian tree and is used on chocolates and sweets to give a glazed and polished look.

E904 Shellac
Shellac is used to glaze sweets and sugary cake decorations. It is a natural additive that comes from an insect found in India called a 'Lac'.

E905 Microcrystalline wax
Used as a glaze and polish on dried fruits, and in sweets, chewing gum and cheese rind, this synthetic wax is made from mineral hydrocarbons.

E912 Montan acid esters
A glazing agent. Permitted to be used on fresh citrus fruits, fresh melon, mango, papaya, avocado and pineapple.

E914 Oxidized polyethylene wax
A glazing agent. Permitted to be used on fresh citrus fruits, fresh melon, mango, papaya, avocado and pineapple.

E920 L-cysteine
This additive is used as a flour improver. It is synthetically produced from the amino acid protein building block called cysteine, and is found in foods like bread.

E927b Carbamide
A flour improver added to bags of bread-making flour to help the dough's fermentation.

E938 Argon
E939 Helium
E941 Nitrogen
E942 Nitrous oxide
E948 Oxygen
E949 Hydrogen
These are packaging gases. They are generally permitted for use in all foods.

E943a Butane
E943b Iso-butane
E944 Propane
These are all propellant gases. Permitted use is limited to vegetable oil, pan sprays and water-based emulsion sprays.

E999 Quillaia extract
A foaming agent. Permitted use is restricted to cider and water-based soft drinks.

E1200 Polydextrose
A bulking agent generally permitted for use in most processed foods.

E1201 Polyvinylpyrrolidone
E1202 Polyvinylpolypyrrolidone
These are both humectants. Permitted use is restricted to tablet and coated tablet dietary food supplements.

E1400-E1414
E1404 Oxidized starch; E1410 Monostarch phosphate; E1412 Distarch phosphate; E1413 Phosphated distarch phosphate; E1414 Acetylated starch. These additives are all starches derived from potato, maize, corn, wheat or tapioca and are used to modify the texture of foods like sauces and chutneys, meat, fish, sweets and baked foods.

E1420 Acetylated starch
E1422 Acetylated distarch adipate
E1440 Hydroxyl propyl starch
E1442 Hydroxy propyl distarch phosphate
E1450 Starch sodium octenyl succinate
E1451 Acetylated oxidized starch
These are all modified starches. They are generally permitted for use in most processed foods.

E1505 Triethyl citrate
This is a stabilizer. Permitted use is restricted to dried egg white.

E1518 Glyceryl triacetate; Triacetin
This is a carrier solvent. Permitted use as glazing agent is restricted to chewing gum.

E1520 Propan-1,2-diol; Propylene glycol
A man-made additive to which flavours and spices are added. It also acts as a stabilizer and humectant and is found in a wide variety of foods.

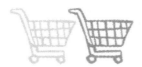

Resource Guide

References

Much of the information in the book came from the following references:

The Food Labelling Regulations 1996, No 1499, HMSO

The Food Labelling (Amendment) (No. 2) Regulations 1999, No. 1483, The Stationery Office

Code of Practice on Health Claims on Foods. Joint Health Claims Initiative

Food Additives Legislation Guidance Notes. Food Standards Agency, March 2002

Nutrition Labelling and Health Claims, British Nutrition Foundation, September 2002

Proposal for a Regulation of the European Parliament and of the Council on Nutrition and Health Claims Made on Foods. 2003/0165 (COD), OJEC

Guidance Notes on Nutrition Labelling, MAFF 1999.

The Genetically Modified & Novel Foods (Labelling) (England) Regulations 2000, The Stationery Office

'This Product May Contain Nuts' Voluntary Labelling Guidelines for Food Allergens and Gluten, Institute of Grocery Distribution, May 2000

Marketing Food to Kids, The Consumers' Association, August 2003

Honest Labelling Campaign, The Consumers' Association, April 2002

Food Labels – The Hidden Truth, The Consumers' Association, July 2002

Useful Contacts
Food Labelling Regulations
www.lhmso.gov.uk/si/si1996/uksi_1996/499_en_l.htm

Food Standards Agency
www.foodstandards.gov.uk

The Consumers' Association
2 Marylebone Road
London NW1 4DF
Tel: 020 7770 7612
www.which.net/campaigns/food

British Nutrition Foundation
High Holborn House
52–54 High Holborn
London WC1V 6RQ
Tel: 020 7404 6504
Email: postbox@nutrition.org.uk

The Institute of Grocery Distribution
Grange Lane
Letchmore Heath
Watford WD2 8DQ
Tel: 01923 857141
www.igd.com
Email: igd@igd.com

Coeliac UK
PO Box No. 220
High Wycombe HP11 2HY
Tel: 01494 437278
www.coeliac.co.uk

The Vegetarian Society
Parkdale
Dunham Road
Altrincham WA14 4QG
Tel: 0161 925 2000
www.vegsoc.org;
Email: info@vegsoc.org

The Vegan Society
Donald Watson House
7 Battle Road
St Leonards-on-Sea TN3 7AA
Tel: 01424 427393
www.vegansociety.com

The Soil Association
Bristol House
40–56 Victoria Street
Bristol BS1 6BY
Tel: 0117 929 0661
www.soilassociation.org
Email: info@soilassociation.org

The National Osteoporosis Society
Camerton
Bath BA2 0PJ
Tel: 01761 471771
www.nos.org.uk
Email: info@nos.org.uk

Diabetes UK
10 Parkway
London NW1 7AA
Tel: 020 7424 1000
www.diabetes.org.uk
Email: info@diabetes.org.uk

HEART UK
7 North Road
Maidenhead SL6 1PE
Tel: 01628 628638

Baby Organix
www.babyorganix.co.uk

Fair Trade
www.fairtrade.org.uk/products.htm

Information on additives
For information on artificial sweeteners, enzymes and
flavourings, please contact:
stephen.knight@foodstandards.gsi.gov.uk
or telephone him on 020 7276 8583

For information on all other additives, please contact:
andy.furmage@foodstandards.gsi.gov.uk
or telephone him on 020 7276 8570

Index

Numbers in *italics* refer to tables.